Digestive Disorders of the Forestomach

Editors

ROBERT J. CALLAN
MEREDYTH L. JONES

VETERINARY CLINICS OF NORTH AMERICA: FOOD ANIMAL PRACTICE

www.vetfood.theclinics.com

Consulting Editor
ROBERT A. SMITH

November 2017 • Volume 33 • Number 3

ELSEVIER

1600 John F. Kennedy Boulevard • Suite 1800 • Philadelphia, Pennsylvania, 19103-2899

http://www.vetfood.theclinics.com

VETERINARY CLINICS OF NORTH AMERICA: FOOD ANIMAL PRACTICE Volume 33, Number 3
November 2017 ISSN 0749-0720, ISBN-13: 978-0-323-54907-3

Editor: Colleen Dietzler
Developmental Editor: Meredith Madeira

Veterinary Clinics of North America: Food Animal Practice (ISSN 0749-0720) is published in March, July, and November by Elsevier Inc., 360 Park Avenue South, New York, NY 10010-1710. Subscription prices are $240.00 per year (domestic individuals), $386.00 per year (domestic institutions), $100.00 per year (domestic students/residents), $265.00 per year (Canadian individuals), $509.00 per year (Canadian institutions), $335.00 per year (international individuals), $509.00 per year (international institutions), and $165.00 per year (international and Canadian students/residents). To receive student/resident rate, orders must be accompanied by name of affiliated institution, date of term, and the signature of program/residency coordinator on institution letterhead. *Clinics* subscription prices. All prices are subject to change without notice. **POSTMASTER:** Send address changes to *Veterinary Clinics of North America*: *Food Animal Practice*, Elsevier Health Sciences Division, Subscription Customer Service, 3251 Riverport Lane, Maryland Heights, MO 63043. Customer Service (orders, claims, online, change of address): Elsevier Health Sciences Division, Subscription **Customer Service, 3251 Riverport Lane, Maryland Heights, MO 63043. Tel: 1-800-654-2452 (U.S. and Canada); 314-447-8871 (ouside U.S. and Canada). Fax: 314-447-8029. E-mail: journalscustomerservice-usa@elsevier.com (for print support); journalsonlinesupport-usa@elsevier.com (for online support).**

Reprints. For copies of 100 or more, of articles in this publication, please contact the Commercial Reprints Department, Elsevier Inc., 360 Park Avenue South, New York, NY 10010-1710. Tel.: 212-633-3874; Fax: 212-633-3820; E-mail: reprints@elsevier.com.

Veterinary Clinics of North America: Food Animal Practice is covered in *Current Contents/Agriculture, Biology and Environmental Sciences, MEDLINE/PubMed (Index Medicus),* and *Excerpta Medica.*

Contributors

CONSULTING EDITOR

ROBERT A. SMITH, DVM, MS
Diplomate, American Board of Veterinary Practitioners; Veterinary Research and Consulting Services, LLC, Greeley, Colorado

EDITORS

ROBERT J. CALLAN, DVM, MS, PhD
Diplomate, American College of Veterinary Internal Medicine; Professor, Livestock Medicine and Surgery, Department of Clinical Sciences, College of Veterinary Medicine and Biomedical Sciences, Colorado State University, Fort Collins, Colorado

MEREDYTH L. JONES, DVM, MS
Associate Professor, Department of Large Animal Clinical Sciences, College of Veterinary Medicine and Biomedical Sciences, Texas A&M University, College Station, Texas

AUTHORS

TANYA J. APPLEGATE, DVM
Senior Resident, Livestock Medicine and Surgery, Department of Clinical Sciences, College of Veterinary Medicine and Biomedical Sciences, Colorado State University, Fort Collins, Colorado

RANSOM L. BALDWIN VI, PhD
Research Animal Scientist, Animal Genomics Improvement Laboratory, Agricultural Research Service, US Department of Agriculture, Beltsville Agricultural Research Center, Beltsville, Maryland

TONY C. BRYANT, MS, PhD
Staff Nutritionist, JBS Five Rivers Cattle Feeding, LLC, Greeley, Colorado; Affiliate Faculty, Department of Animal Sciences, Colorado State University, Fort Collins, Colorado

ROBERT J. CALLAN, DVM, MS, PhD
Diplomate, American College of Veterinary Internal Medicine; Professor, Livestock Medicine and Surgery, Department of Clinical Sciences, College of Veterinary Medicine and Biomedical Sciences, Colorado State University, Fort Collins, Colorado

ERIN E. CONNOR, PhD
Research Molecular Biologist, Animal Genomics Improvement Laboratory, Agricultural Research Service, US Department of Agriculture, Beltsville Agricultural Research Center, Beltsville, Maryland

BRENT CREDILLE, DVM, PhD
Diplomate, American College of Veterinary Internal Medicine; Assistant Professor, Section Head, Food Animal Health and Management Program, Department of Population Health, University of Georgia College of Veterinary Medicine, Veterinary Medical Center, Athens, Georgia

AHMED A. ELOLIMY, MS
PhD candidate, Department of Animal Sciences, Division of Nutritional Sciences, University of Illinois, Urbana, Illinois

DEREK FOSTER, DVM, PhD
Diplomate, American College of Veterinary Internal Medicine-Large Animal; Assistant Professor of Ruminant Medicine, Department of Population Health and Pathobiology, NC State College of Veterinary Medicine, Raleigh, North Carolina

JUAN J. LOOR, PhD
Associate Professor, Department of Animal Sciences, Division of Nutritional Sciences, University of Illinois, Urbana, Illinois

JOSHUA C. McCANN, PhD
Assistant Professor, Department of Animal Sciences, Division of Nutritional Sciences, University of Illinois, Urbana, Illinois

NATHAN F. MEYER, MS, MBA, PhD, DVM
Staff Nutritionist and Veterinarian, JBS Five Rivers Cattle Feeding, LLC, Greeley, Colorado; Affiliate Faculty, Department of Clinical Sciences, Colorado State University, Fort Collins, Colorado

MATT D. MIESNER, DVM, MS
Associate Clinical Professor, Veterinary Clinical Sciences, Kansas State University, Manhattan, Kansas

DUSTY W. NAGY, DVM, MS, PhD
Department of Veterinary Medicine and Surgery, University of Missouri, College of Veterinary Medicine, Columbia, Missouri

GARRETT R. OETZEL, DVM, MS
Professor, Food Animal Production Medicine Section, Department of Medical Sciences, School of Veterinary Medicine, University of Wisconsin - Madison, Madison, Wisconsin

EMILY J. REPPERT, DVM, MS
Assistant Professor, Veterinary Clinical Sciences, Kansas State University, Manhattan, Kansas

EMILY SNYDER, DVM, MFAM
Graduate Assistant, Food Animal Health and Management Program, Department of Population Health, University of Georgia College of Veterinary Medicine, Veterinary Medical Center, Athens, Georgia

Contents

> The ruminal epithelium is a complex tissue that serves as an important protective barrier as well as a metabolically important tissue for whole-animal energy metabolism. Up to 70% of the energetic needs of mature animals are absorbed as short-chain fatty acids through the stratified squamous epithelium, and it serves as the primary producer of ketones in fed animals. Both physical and metabolic development are incomplete at birth and are triggered by short-chain fatty acids. Regulatory control of the proliferation and differentiation necessary for normal development is a useful model for the scientific investigation of nutrient-gene interactions.

 Video content accompanies this article at http://www.vetfood. theclinics.com.

> Primary diseases of the forestomach are caused by disruptions in the ruminal wall and contraction cycle or by a disruption in the normal flora and fermentation processes. Secondary disease of the reticulorumen is caused by abnormalities in rumen contraction and/or fermentation secondary to other systemic illnesses. Rumen function is complex, and the contraction cycle and fermentation are interrelated, which allows for overlapping results in diagnostic tests. Physical examination, combined with diagnostic tests such as rumen fluid analysis, radiography, and ultrasonography, can be used to categorize and diagnose ruminant forestomach disease.

> Clinical rumen acidosis is an important cause of morbidity and mortality in both large and small ruminants. Feeding and management practices that lead to the consumption of large amounts of readily fermentable carbohydrates precipitate clinical disease. The fermentation of carbohydrates into volatile fatty acids and lactate causes acidosis (local and systemic), rumen ulceration, cardiovascular compromise, and organ dysfunction. Animals affected with acidosis can suffer from numerous sequelae. Treatment of animals with clinical rumen acidosis is focused on addressing plasma volume deficits, correcting acid-base disturbances, and restoring a normal rumen microenvironment.

Subacute ruminal acidosis (SARA) is a common problem in lactating dairy cows that causes chronic health problems, impairs feed efficiency, and increases the environmental impact of milk production. Low ruminal pH appears to be the main instigator of the pathophysiology of SARA, although other metabolites produced in the rumen may be involved. Inflammatory responses to SARA are variable but important determinants of a cow's response to SARA. SARA can be diagnosed at the herd level by integrating information about clinical signs and on-farm measures of ruminal pH. Prevention of SARA requires excellent feeding management and proper diet formulation.

Ruminal acidosis and ruminal bloat represent the most common digestive disorders in feedlot cattle. Ruminants are uniquely adapted to digest and metabolize a large range of feedstuffs. Although cattle have the ability to handle various feedstuffs, disorders associated with altered ruminal fermentation can occur. Proper ruminal microorganism adaptation and a consistent substrate (ration) help prevent digestive disorders. Feed bunk management, sufficient ration fiber, consistent feed milling, and appropriate response to abnormal weather are additional factors important in prevention of digestive disorders. When digestive disorders are suspected, timely diagnosis is imperative.

Rumen distension and hypomotility are common clinical findings in ruminants. A thorough physical examination to assess the rumen shape and consistency of rumen contents are critical to determining the underlying pathology. Most cases can be classified into 1 of the 4 types of vagal indigestion. Type 1 is characterized by gas distension of the rumen dorsally on the left side. Types 2, 3, and 4 will often appear similar on physical examination with fluid distension of the rumen on the left and ventrally on the right. Serum chloride and bicarbonate measurement and assessment of rumen chloride allow for differentiation of type 2 versus types 3 and 4 vagal indigestion. This is critical, as type 2 vagal indigestion will commonly require a rumenotomy, whereas types 3 and 4 typically are addressed through a right flank exploratory.

 Video content accompanies this article at http://www.vetfood. theclinics.com.

Eating habits in cattle are less discriminant than other ruminants, and they more often accidentally ingest strange objects while feeding. Penetrating foreign bodies may cause mild to severe peritonitis, penetrate the diaphragm to cause pleuritis or pericarditis, or cause localized abscesses in the thorax or abdomen. Because these objects are most often metal, a common term for this problem is hardware disease. An accurate history and thorough physical examination often yields a diagnosis; however, ancillary diagnostics can enhance accuracy and disease magnitude before exploratory surgery. Treatment encompasses controlling infection and inflammation and foreign body removal; preventive measures are emphasized.

Temporary rumenostomy is a useful procedure for the treatment, management, and support of patients with forestomach disease of various types. The rumenostomy provides a mechanism for relief of chronic rumen tympany or distention, removal of rumen contents and lavage of the rumen, removal of some rumen foreign bodies, administration of rumen fluid transfaunation, and administration of enteral nutrition or other medications. When the rumenostomy is no longer necessary, it can be allowed to close by second intention or by surgical resection.

Fermentation of a variety of feedstuffs by the ruminal microbiome is the distinctive feature of the ruminant digestive tract. The host derives energy and nutrients from microbiome activity; these organisms are essential to survival. Advances in DNA sequencing and bioinformatics have redefined the rumen microbial community. Current research seeks to connect our understanding of the rumen microbiome with nutritional strategies in ruminant livestock systems and their associated digestive disorders. These efforts align with a growing number of products designed to improve ruminal fermentation to benefit the overall efficiency of ruminant livestock production and health.

VETERINARY CLINICS OF NORTH AMERICA: FOOD ANIMAL PRACTICE

THE CLINICS ARE NOW AVAILABLE ONLINE!
Access your subscription at:
www.theclinics.com

Preface

Digestive Disorders of the Ruminant Forestomach

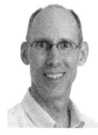
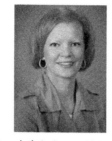

Robert J. Callan, DVM, MS, PhD   Meredyth L. Jones, DVM, MS
Editors

When presented with the proposal to edit a *Veterinary Clinics of North America: Food Animal Practice* issue on Digestive Disorders of Ruminants, the request seemed both exciting and daunting. A review of previous issues dating back to 1986 showed that an issue of similar topic was absent, the closest being Diagnosis of Digestive Diseases, in March 2000. The scope of the topics covering digestive disorders of ruminants is immense, and it was readily apparent that a single issue would not suffice. Thankfully, Elsevier agreed to divide this topic into two issues, the present focusing on Forestomach Disorders, and a following issue, Digestive Disorders of the Ruminant Abomasum and Intestines.

The ruminant forestomach is a remarkable anatomic and physiologic organ that allows ruminants the ability to digest various forms of forages and grains through microbial fermentation. Appropriate forestomach function, digestion, and nutrient absorption are dependent on the proper interrelations of anatomic development, physiological environment, microbial populations, and motor activity. Given the complexity of these processes, forestomach disease is a very common clinical presentation that can be challenging to localize, diagnose, and effectively treat. The goal of this issue is to provide food animal practitioners with the most up-to-date information to help evaluate and treat the individual animal and manage herd health problems relevant to ruminant forestomach physiology, microbiology, and common medical disorders. We were fortunate to obtain some of the top researchers and clinicians in the field to provide these in-depth reviews of relevant topics, including forestomach development, microbiology, diagnostic evaluation, diseases, and treatment.

These clinical reviews demonstrate that our understanding and application of physiology, nutrition, microbiology, diagnostics, and medical intervention of forestomach disorders continue to progress. Utilization of new technology and concepts complements the clinical practices that have stood the test of time. Better understanding of

Vet Clin Food Anim 33 (2017) ix–x
http://dx.doi.org/10.1016/j.cvfa.2017.06.010
0749-0720/17/© 2017 Published by Elsevier Inc.

vetfood.theclinics.com

forestomach development and the role of nutrition in supporting cellular function and nutrient utilization provide effective management tools to improve health and production efficiency. The microbial environment plays a critical role in forestomach function; however, we are only beginning to understand the complex diversity of the forestomach microbial population through the use of modern genomic techniques. The ability to manipulate the forestomach microbiome has tremendous implications for future health and productivity of ruminants. Various probiotics and feed additives are available to promote and maintain forestomach health and are likely to become more common as our knowledge and evidence of benefits grow. Even with our current ability to promote a healthy rumen microflora, rumen acidosis continues to be a major health issue on both an individual and a herd scale in dairy and beef feedlot operations. Also included in this issue are articles focused on the diagnostic approach to forestomach disorders, evaluation and interpretation of forestomach motility disorders, evaluation and treatment of hardware disease, and the use of temporary rumenostomy for treating forestomach disorders.

It is our hope that this issue will broaden the practicing clinician's understanding of forestomach physiology, function, and microbiology and provide useful approaches to the diagnosis, treatment, and prevention of common forestomach disorders.

Robert J. Callan, DVM, MS, PhD
Department of Clinical Sciences
College of Veterinary Medicine and Biomedical Sciences
Colorado State University
300 West Drake Road
Fort Collins, CO 80523-1678, USA

Meredyth L. Jones, DVM, MS
Department of Large Animal Clinical Sciences
College of Veterinary Medicine and Biomedical Sciences
Texas A&M University
4475 TAMU
College Station, TX 77843, USA

E-mail addresses:
Robert.Callan@ColoState.edu (R.J. Callan)
MJones@cvm.tamu.edu (M.L. Jones)

Rumen Function and Development

Ransom L. Baldwin VI, PhD*, Erin E. Connor, PhD

KEYWORDS

- Rumen • Epithelium • Metabolism • Development • Differentiation

KEY POINTS

- Rumen epithelial character and composition are unique among other gastrointestinal tissues that serve both protective and metabolic functions of critical importance to productive ruminants.
- Rumen epithelial development is incomplete at birth and requires the establishment of ruminal fermentation, and the production of short-chain fatty acids (the most potent is butyrate) to initiate the maturation processes.
- Metabolic and physical adaptations occur simultaneously and result in altered production efficiency, depending on dietary composition.
- Regulatory control in response to butyrate seems to be a result of both proliferative and metabolism-specific adaptations driven by differential expression of key regulatory genes.

INTRODUCTION

The ruminal epithelium is uniquely placed to affect the net use of nutrients of the whole body. The symbiosis between the microbiome inhabiting the lumen and the host largely depends on the provision of a constant supply of nutrients from roughage that would otherwise be unusable to the mammalian digestive system. Physically a barrier to the contents of the lumen, the rumen epithelium serves an obvious protective function, which, when compromised, results in disease states. The ruminal epithelium is a stratified squamous epithelium which are typically associated with protective functions rather than absorption. As such, ruminal epithelium is unlike other gastrointestinal tissue barriers. Metabolically, the ruminal lining serves a critical role in

Disclosure: The authors have nothing to disclose.
Disclaimer: Mention of a product, reagent, or source does not constitute an endorsement by the US Department of Agriculture (USDA) to the exclusion of other products or services that perform a comparable function. The USDA is an equal opportunity provider and employer.
Animal Genomics Improvement Laboratory, Agricultural Research Service, US Department of Agriculture, Beltsville Agricultural Research Center, 10300 Baltimore Avenue, Beltsville, MD 20705, USA
* Corresponding author.
E-mail address: ransom.baldwin@ars.usda.gov

mitigating the diffusion of end products of fermented feedstuffs into circulation. The metabolic contributions of the ruminal epithelium have received a great deal of research attention because the impact of the tissue on production efficiency is undeniable. Moreover, the process and regulation of the developing rumen epithelium has received a great deal of research interest because the tissue is incompletely developed at birth and requires the establishment of a viable ruminal fermentation for complete development by weaning. This developmental process has been viewed with interest not only from the health and well-being aspect of rearing replacement heifers and production animals but also as a unique model system for the investigation of nutrient-gene interactions occurring naturally. This article describes the basic structure and metabolic characteristics of the epithelial lining of the rumen, and discusses the importance of the differentiation of the tissue during normal development production practices.

IMPORTANCE OF GASTROINTESTINAL TISSUES TO PRODUCTION EFFICIENCY

The gastrointestinal tract has a large impact on the nutrient economy of the whole animal by virtue of its critical position in the process and the large cost of nutrient extraction from feedstuffs required before delivery of metabolites to the productive tissues (ie, mammary gland, muscle). Thus, production-oriented research has been interested in these tissues and their contribution to the maintenance requirements. From a metabolic standpoint, maintenance functions of the visceral organs primarily include Na^+-/K^+-ATPase activity, protein synthesis and degradation, substrate cycling, and urea synthesis.[1] The ruminant gastrointestinal tract as a whole is responsible for 40% of the whole- body ATP use.[1] In addition, a simulation of protein turnover in growing lambs predicts that 19% of total-body ATP expenditure is caused by protein turnover and that 25% to 27% is caused by gastrointestinal tract protein turnover.[2] Because of these aforementioned energetic and nutrient costs, the maintenance of the gastrointestinal tract tissues in growing ruminants has an extensive impact on whole-body metabolism. However, in production settings, defining the cost of the gut tissues is complicated by the mass of these tissues changing in response to plane of nutrition, dietary chemical composition, and the physiologic status of the animal.[3–6] It has been generally observed that cell-specific or mass-specific changes in metabolism are largely unaffected by plane of nutrition.[7–10] However, as discussed later, dietary composition and nutrient delivery to the tissue do affect metabolism, and, thus, understanding both proliferative and metabolic control is necessary for accurate prediction of nutrient use efficiency.

STRUCTURE AND FUNCTION OF THE RUMINAL EPITHELIUM IN MATURE RUMINANTS

Rumen epithelium provides several physiologically vital functions, including absorption, transport, volatile fatty acid metabolism, and protection.[11,12] The ruminal epithelium is a stratified squamous epithelium consisting of 4 strata: stratum basale, stratum spinosum, stratum granulosum, and stratum corneum (**Fig. 1**).[13,14] Cell layers vary within each stratum and vary starkly depending on diet, stage of ruminal development, and feeding pattern. The cells of the stratum basale, adjacent to the basal lamina, contain fully functional mitochondria and other organelles, and are the cells of the rumen that contribute most significantly to the metabolic properties of the tissue (ie, ketogenesis). Ketogenic enzymes are principally located within the mitochondria of the ruminal epithelium. Consequently, basale cells are likely the most important ruminal layer relative to the energy metabolism of the whole animal.[15] The stratum spinosum and stratum granulosum are the intermediate cell layers and are not separated

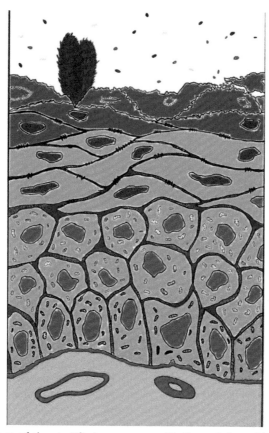

Fig. 1. The structure of the stratified squamous epithelium of the epithelial lining of the rumen. (*Adapted from* Steele MA, Penner GB, Chaucheyras-Durand F, et al. Development and physiology of the rumen and the lower gut: targets for improving gut health. J Dairy Sci 2016;99:4956; with permission.)

by a distinct division.[16] As the cells migrate through these intermediate layers they contain progressively fewer mitochondria, and take on a less uniform appearance. In the stratum granulosum the cells have established tight gap junctions (desmosomes) that maintain the integrity of metabolite concentration gradients across the rumen wall.[12,13] Cells in the stratum corneum, the most exposed cell strata, are highly cornified, and presumably function as a defensive barrier against the physical environment of the rumen. The desmosomal integrity of the stratum corneum is degenerated and large gaps exist between individual cells.[13,14] Dietary composition, and thus ruminal environment, greatly affects the number of cell layers present in the stratum corneum.[14–17] For example, production rations high in concentrate decrease ruminal pH, increase propionate/acetate ratios, and increase molar proportions of butyrate, which can result in a 15-cell-layer thickness in the stratum corneum.[17] In contrast, animals maintained on a predominantly roughage diet often have stratum corneum consisting of as few as 4 cell layers.[17] Although feeding regimen (ie, how and when the feed is presented) has been implicated as affecting the stratum corneum,[16,18] these adaptations are more likely attributable to the subsequent alterations in the ruminal environment.[11]

METABOLISM OF MATURE RUMINAL EPITHELIUM

The rumen and reticulum account for more than 70% of the total digestive tract volume by weight.[19] Vast numbers of papillae protrude from the ruminal surface into the lumen, greatly increasing the surface area available for absorption of volatile fatty acids or short-chain fatty acids (SCFAs).[20] Most (>75%)[21] of the SCFAs are absorbed through the epithelial lining of the rumen and reticulum, with less than 10% of the ruminally produced SCFAs reaching the small intestine.[20] Rate and capacity for SCFA removal from the ruminal lumen is influenced by the pH of the rumen contents. Specifically, when ruminal pH is near neutrality (7.2), all of the SCFAs are absorbed at similar rates. When ruminal pH decreases o less than 6.0, the rate of SCFA absorption declines concomitantly.[22] In particular, reduction in acetate and propionate absorption is more sensitive to decreases in pH than butyrate. Thus, at low ruminal pH, butyrate absorption increases as a proportion of total SCFAs absorbed, but the absorption rate remains less than that observed at near-neutral pH.[17,22] However, the ruminal epithelium is not simply a barrier to nutrient diffusion but acts to maintain the integrity of metabolite concentration gradients through the metabolism of primarily butyrate, and other SCFAs. Acetate, propionate, and butyrate are metabolized to different extents by the ruminal epithelium. In addition, ruminal SCFA metabolism protects against potentially detrimental decreases in blood pH.[17]

VOLATILE FATTY ACID METABOLISM
Acetate

Acetate is present in the rumen in the highest concentrations of all of the SCFAs produced by the rumen microbes. Acetate is used for fat synthesis by the adipose tissue and as an energy substrate by all extrahepatic tissues of the animal. Appearance of acetate in portal blood is highly correlated with acetate concentration within the ruminal lumen.[22,23] The absorption of acetate increases with ruminal development and decreases in response to high-concentrate diets,[24] presumably caused by decreases in ruminal pH and acetate/propionate ratio. In vitro experiments indicate that acetate is absorbed readily by the ruminal epithelia.[25] However, acetate addition fails to induce an increase in oxygen uptake by rumen tissue slices,[25] indicating that the tissue does not metabolize acetate to a great extent. However, acetate causes a decrease in butyrate conversion to β-hydroxybutyrate (βHBA) production,[15] which is likely attributed to acetyl coenzyme A (CoA) formation and a net inhibition of butyryl-CoA synthesis, and thereby decreased butyrate metabolism. Regardless, the extent to which acetate was oxidized to CO_2 was minimal in those same experiments.[15]

Propionate

Propionate is the primary gluconeogenic substrate used by ruminant liver and can account for 60% of the glucose used by the animal.[20] Propionate seems to undergo limited metabolism to lactate and pyruvate by the ruminal epithelium.[26,27] Estimates range from 3% to 15% of absorbed propionate undergoing metabolism, primarily to lactate and pyruvate.[24,27,28] In vitro, propionate induces no change in oxygen uptake by rumen pieces.[25] Despite the apparently low use of propionate by the ruminal epithelium, disappearance of propionate-derived carbon from the rumen cannot be completely accounted for by the concentrations of lactate, pyruvate, and propionate appearing in the portal blood.[23] Moreover, in isolated rumen epithelial cell preparations, propionate metabolism affects butyrate metabolism.[29] These changes are likely caused by changing redox status in the cells dictating net output of ketone bodies in the form of acetoacetate versus βHBA.

Propionate activation to propionyl-CoA by propionyl-CoA synthetase is the limiting step in propionate metabolism.[26] Propionyl-CoA synthetase activity is sensitive to the developmental state of the rumen and to the molar proportion of propionate in the ruminal fluid.[24,26] Following activation to propionyl-CoA, the propionate-derived carbon is converted to methyl-malonyl-CoA and subsequently enters the TCA (tricarboxylic acid) cycle as succinyl-CoA. Propionate metabolism to lactate and pyruvate may serve to maintain the balance of cytosolic nicotinamide adenine dinucleotide (NAD)/NAD, reduced form (NADH) in the ruminal epithelium of concentrate-fed animals.[28] Metabolism of propionate to lactate and pyruvate may also result in preservation of propionate-derived carbon for gluconeogenesis, because the liver quantitatively removes pyruvate and lactate from the portal blood.[23]

Butyrate

Unlike nonruminants, in which ketone bodies (βHBA and acetoacetate [AcAc]) are used as a last resort during hypoglycemia (usually starvation conditions), ketone bodies are continuously used as an energy source by the extrahepatic tissues of the ruminant animal, and, in the fed animal, rumen and liver are the primary producers of ketone bodies.[30] Ruminally derived AcAc is quantitatively removed from portal blood by the liver and metabolized to βHBA. Thus, in the fed state, the ruminal epithelium is the primary source of circulating ketone bodies in ruminant animals. Most (85%–90%) of ruminally absorbed butyrate-derived carbon appearing in portal blood is in the form of βHBA and AcAc.[31] The balance of the absorbed butyrate-derived carbon can be accounted for as CO_2 produced as a result of oxidation.[25]

Ketogenesis in the ruminal epithelium occurs exclusively in the mitochondria because of the compartmentalization of the ketogenic enzymes.[32] Two pathways of ketogenesis are available to the ruminal epithelium. Ketogenesis can progress through 3-hydroxy-3-methylglutaryl-CoA (HMG-CoA) synthase and HMG-CoA lyase (as in the liver) or via deacylation of AcAc-CoA catalyzed by succinyl-CoA transferase. Both of these pathways result in the production of AcAc. The final step in ruminal ketogenesis is the production of βHBA catalyzed by βHBA dehydrogenase. In fed ruminants, this pathway is favored because of the NADH/NAD ratio of the mitochondria.[30] All of these ketogenic enzymes are present within the ruminal epithelium at sufficient activity levels to account for the ketogenic capacity of the rumen.[32,33]

Rumen development
Morphologic observations It is well established that the rumen is incompletely developed both physically and metabolically at birth.[34] In neonates, the rumen does not show the high degree of keratinization characteristic of the mature organ[35]; metabolically, the rumen is essentially nonfunctional with respect to ketogenic capacity.[36] Following the initiation of solid feed intake by the neonate and the subsequent establishment of the ruminal fermentation, the rumen undergoes both physical and metabolic development. Physical development of the rumen can be further partitioned into 2 aspects: increases in rumen mass, and growth of the papillae (**Fig. 2**). Early research indicated that physical stimulation by feed in the rumen could account for measurable increases in both rumen weight and musculature development. However, the presence of physical bulk does not promote papillary development.[37] Thus, for normal development of the ruminal epithelium to progress, a viable ruminal fermentation must be established, suggesting that there is a requirement for the presence of SCFA in the ruminal lumen to promote normal papillary development.[38]

Compared with grain-fed and hay-fed control animals, neonatal ruminants maintained solely on milk during the first months of life show limited ruminal development with

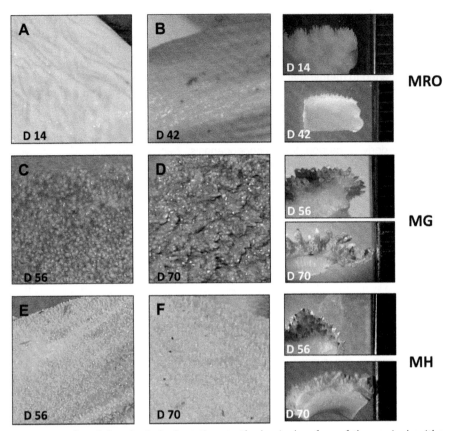

Fig. 2. Examples of the physical adaptations to the luminal surface of the ruminal epithe-lium when exposed to different dietary regimens: milk replacer only (MRO), milk replacer to 42 days then weaned onto calf starter (MG), milk replacer to 42 days then weaned onto orchard grass hay (MH) at 4 stages of development. (*A*) MRO-fed calf at 14 days (D 14) of age. (*B*) MRO-fed calf at 42 days of age. (*C*) MG-fed calf at 56 d of age (*D*) MG-fed calf at 70 days of age (*E*) MH-fed calf at 56 days of age (*F*) MH-fed calf at 70 days of age. Note that magnification of the large panels is not uniform for the high-magnification panels on the right. A scale bar is included in 1-mm increments. (*From* Connor EE, Baldwin RL, Li C, et al. Gene expression in bovine rumen epithelium during weaning identifies molecular regulators of rumen development and growth. Funct Integr Genomics 2013;13:137; with permission.)

respect to rumen weight,[39–42] capacity,[39,43] papillary growth,[34,39,41] degree of keratini-zation,[35] pigmentation,[39] and musculature development.[37,39,43] The lack of develop-ment in the absence of solid feed intake is likely caused by the effective shunting of milk directly to the abomasum by the reflexive closure of the esophageal groove,[44] thus preventing substrate to support the establishment of a ruminal fermentation from entering the rumen. Consistent with this, when milk is infused directly into the rumen, resulting in SCFA production, papillary growth is stimulated.[39] Also, direct ruminal infu-sion of SCFA (50% of estimated net energy requirement) at physiologic concentrations similarly results in increases in papillae length in lambs.[40] In contrast, use of ruminally inert materials such as nylon bristles, plastic sponges, wood shavings, and plastic cubes to simulate the physical stimulus of feed in the rumen resulted in no significant papillary development.[34,37,39,43] Infusions of sodium salts of propionate and butyrate, but not acetate, chloride, or glucose, resulted in marked development of the ruminal papillae in calves.[38,39] Similarly, a mixture of SCFA salts (propionate and butyrate included) fed as 10% (weight/weight) of a concentrate starter ration resulted in increased incidence of ruminal parakeratosis, and in all treated animals a thickening of the stratum corneum was reported in calves[35] and lambs.[45] Increasing amounts of concentrate in the diet resulted in no change in rumen muscularity but did result in increased papillae density and papillae height in calves[19,41] and lambs.[45] None of these early studies were able to definitively distinguish the mechanism responsible for the induction of papillary development. However, all added to the recognition of butyrate as a putative nutrient that regulates differentiation and proliferation of the mammalian tissue.

Control of Proliferation Ruminal epithelial cell proliferation has been evaluated with both in vivo[46–49] and in vitro[50] by measuring ^{3}H-thymidine incorporation and mitotic indices. Butyric acid infused directly into the rumen of sheep resulted in a stimulation of mitotic indices.[46,47] In a series of similar trials, a single pulse dose of sodium butyrate followed by continuous saline infusion stimulated mitotic indices to a greater extent than a pulse-chase regimen with sodium butyrate. Thus, a rapid but unsustained increase in butyrate level in the rumen, which is not observed physiologically, stimulates cell proliferation. Similarly, although to a lesser extent, both propionate and acetate were also stimulatory when administered as a single dose.[49]

In contrast with the in vivo findings, cellular DNA incorporation of ^{3}H-thymidine by isolated ruminal epithelial cells is decreased in a dose-dependent manner by sodium butyrate in the medium.[50] Explant cultures were further used to show that butyrate arrests cell division near the basal lamina while increasing the keratinization and protein expression of the other cell types. The net result is an increase in both size and cornification of the explant.[11] Isolated cells in culture treated with butyrate similarly showed decreased proliferation.[51] The apparent differences in the in vivo and in vitro responses, and the seemingly contradictory nature of the in vivo reports, suggest an indirect pathway of cell stimulation. Ruminal epithelial mitotic indices have been shown to be stimulated by intravenous insulin infusions[52] and because propionate has been shown to stimulate insulin release in vivo[52] it was theorized that insulin could be a humoral mediator in the stimulation of mitosis in the ruminal epithelium. However, administration of a host of hormones, including pentagastrin, insulin, and glucagon, to isolated ruminal cells all resulted in stimulation of cell proliferation, whereas responses to cortisol were inconsistent.[48,49,52,53] Insulin uniquely overcame the inhibitory effects of butyrate in isolated cells of the stratum basale.[11,53] This finding was extended to epidermal growth factor (EGF) and insulinlike growth factor I (IGF-I), which stimulated cell proliferation rates to 97% and 96%, respectively, of that observed in positive controls treated with 5% fetal calf serum, which has a myriad of growth factors present.[51] Most importantly, the inhibitory action of 1 mM butyrate in vitro was completely overcome by the addition of IGF-I and EGF, and to a lesser extent by insulin. Thus, factors other than direct action by nutrients cannot be wholly eliminated as putative agents controlling ruminal epithelial proliferation, although the regulation by these factors has not yet been delineated conclusively. Metabolic adaptation is likewise of great interest in production as young ruminants are weaned from milk to solid feedstuffs.

Neonatal ruminal epithelial metabolism
The primary source of energetic substrates for rumen epithelium in milk-fed ruminants is derived from intestinally absorbed nutrients rather than nutrients absorbed through the rumen wall, because of the reflexive closure of the esophageal groove and the lack

of SCFAs in the ruminal lumen.[14] Fatty acids and glucose absorbed in the small intestine must first pass through the liver, so it has been assumed that glucose is a primary energy substrate of the immature rumen epithelial tissue (eg, before active fermentation in the lumen), as is the case with other neonatal tissues.[54] Early experiments in vitro evaluated rates of oxygen uptake by rumen slices from 14-day-old calf ruminal epithelium (undeveloped) or mature ruminal papillae in the presence of various oxidizable substrates such as glucose, butyrate, and lactate.[36] Oxygen uptake by the neonatal rumen is greatest when glucose, and to a lesser degree lactate, is present as the oxidizable substrate; however, oxygen consumption by mature rumen papillae increases to more than the basal oxygen uptake when glucose is added, but does not respond as dramatically as neonatal rumen slices.[36,42] In contrast, butyrate stimulates oxygen uptake to a greater degree in mature rumen papillae and isolated cells than in the neonatal rumen. It seems that, under normal weaning production practices, glucose is used as the primary oxidizable energy substrate of the rumen tissues from birth until weaning.[42] However, after weaning, this capacity is greatly decreased, and glucose oxidation by mature ruminal cells decreases to less than that observed in newborn lambs.[42] Butyrate oxidation showed a similar pattern. Initially, rates of oxidation were low followed by high rates of oxidation from 7 days through weaning. Both butyrate and glucose oxidation rates decreased in the presence of the other oxidizable substrates, suggesting a flexibility in oxidative metabolism. Thus, although the ruminal epithelium can use glucose and butyrate as its energetic substrate, neither seems to be the favored substrate. Ketogenesis from butyrate as a substrate is substantially lower in the neonatal rumen compared with the mature tissue, showing a 8-fold increase in βHBA production.[42] Metabolic development is greatly affected when ruminants are reared in the absence of solid feed intake.[55] However, ruminal ketogenesis shows the characteristic marked increase in ketogenic capacity at 42 days regardless of dietary regimen, whereas other metabolic parameters do not follow the normal rearing development characteristics. This finding indicates that an ontogenic response rather than a nutrient-triggered event may also be controlling tissue differentiation. This possibility is supported by an increase in gene transcripts for HMG-CoA synthase (enzyme code [EC] 4.1.3.5),[56] despite the lack of solid feed intake and SCFA production in the rumen. Despite the extensive evidence implicating butyrate as the putative trigger for physical development and metabolic differentiation, ontological control of some of the critical metabolic changes occurring in ruminants cannot be eliminated as a causative factor. These processes can likewise be occurring simultaneously, and further study will be required to fully understand this regulation.

Underlying molecular responses in support of development and function

With the advent of enhanced capacity to evaluate the mechanisms of action at the molecular level, developmental changes have been evaluated at the gene expression level of integration. Temporal responses in gene expression to increased butyrate concentrations of the rumen epithelium using serial biopsy sampling from cows ruminally infused with butyrate for 7 days combined with high-throughput RNA-sequencing technology and bioinformatic tools have been evaluated. In the mature rumen, initial reaction of the rumen epithelium transcriptome to increased exogenous butyrate levels may represent a stress response because gene ontology terms identified as enriched were predominantly related to biological processes, such as response to bacteria and biotic stimuli. Butyrate induced at least 16 tight junction–related genes in in vitro studies, showing the importance of maintaining a physical barrier to diffusion of the rumen.[57] A strong upregulation of major macromolecular components, such as claudins (*CLDN1*, *CLDN3*, *CLDN4*, *CLDN7*, *CLDN12*, and *CLDN23*), tight junction protein 3 (*TJP3*), and junctional adhesion molecules 2 and 3 (*JAM2* and *JAM3*), by butyrate supports the contention that these genes may play an important role in maintaining and/or restoring intestinal barrier function, and that SCFA concentration in the lumen is affecting tissue-specific functions.[57] Moreover, it has been shown that regulatory networks, putatively controlled by transcription factors and mediated by butyrate, are involved in distinct tissue functions, that including solute transport and enzymes affecting SCFA and intermediary metabolism.[57] Another putative activated transcription factor alpha (PPAR-alpha) important to the control of gene expression in weaning animals was identified from characterization of the gene expression changes occurring in weaning calves.[41] In addition, downstream gene targets of PPAR-alpha were responsive to the transition from milk replacer to solid feed in developing calf rumen epithelium. In this case, most of the genes identified participate in oxidation of lipids; however, other functions include apoptosis, organ development, nutrient metabolism, and the immune response. Thus strong evidence exists of the role of nutrients in control of tissue growth, metabolism, and differentiation. However, it does not seem that expression of *PPAR-alpha* messenger RNA is affected by SCFA concentration in bovine rumen,[58] although it seems that SCFAs do interact with PPAR-ligand in the colon.[59] Metabolism-specific changes are also linked to PPAR-alpha pathway because mitochondrial acetyl-CoA acetyltransferase (ACAT1) and mitochondrial hydroxymethylglutaryl-CoA synthase (HMGCS2), which function in metabolic organ development, were upregulated during weaning. The products of these genes play a crucial role in ketogenesis by the rumen epithelium of sheep during development.[56] Furthermore, *ACAT* expression has been shown to be increased in mature rumen epithelium in heifers fed high-concentrate versus low-concentrate diets.[60] Combined, these observations support the hypothesis that increased production of SCFA in response to introduction of solid feed during weaning may promote ketogenesis in rumen epithelium. Thus, although dramatic changes in mature tissue gene expression are often muted or not observed, changes seen in the developmental model serve to elucidate the mechanisms involved in the control of metabolism in the mature differentiated tissue during critical changes in metabolic demand, such as lactation.

An additional area of obvious importance to the role of the ruminal epithelium as a service function tissue in the ruminant is nutrient transport. Changes in specific transporter activity have been recognized, specifically those functioning in SCFA and ion transport of ruminants fed high-concentrate[60] or high-protein[61] diets. A large number of transport-related genes, including the water channel protein *aquaporin 5, copper transport protein*, the intestinal proton-dependent peptide transporter *adherin 17, chloride channel 2, sodium channel (non–voltage-gated 1, gamma subunit), transient receptor potential cation channel (subfamily M, member 6)*, and 20 different solute carrier (*SLC*) family members changed in response to weaning from milk to either forage-based or concentrate-based rations.[41] However, these changes were not always consistent in direction, with upregulation of some (*SLC14A1*, *SLC16A1*, and *SLC26A3*) and downregulation in others (*SLC4A4*). Ontological-based changes in expression of these same genes as well as other transporters occur with age rather than diet.[61] Complete understanding of the transcriptome regulation is still not established with certainty. This exciting area of research clearly needs additional study for elucidation of the impact of dietary changes and rumen developmental changes relating to control of rumen epithelial metabolism.

SUMMARY

Rumen epithelium is responsible for important protective functions, including guarding the host from insult of symbiotic microorganisms inhabiting the lumen, as well as the end products of feedstuff digestion. The character and composition of the tissue are distinct from other digestive tissues, and continued study is needed to clarify the process of rumen development and to elucidate the differential expression of key regulatory processes to better manage the health and well-being of the whole animal. Current approaches have not yet sufficiently separated the critical regulatory pathways influencing the ontological responses, the direct nutrient-gene interactions, or indirect control via endocrine factors. In productive and growing ruminants, dietary effects (ie, energy intake and dietary energy density) on ruminal mass clearly alter protein and energy maintenance requirements in the production setting. However, it is unclear whether these changes in gut mass affect digestive and absorptive capacities. Rumen epithelial metabolism of SCFAs and the role of SCFAs in the stimulation and control of tissue differentiation has clear implications for the digestive capabilities and supply of substrates to growing and mature ruminants. Recent studies focused on transcriptomic changes and epigenetic modifications show that entire gene families are affected by the nutrient delivery system present in the functioning ruminant. Because SCFA concentrations in the neonatal rumen are rarely found at the high levels that occur in mature ruminants, rumen development and maturation have and will continue to serve as a unique model to enhance the understanding of complex control systems.

REFERENCES

1. McBride BW, Kelly JM. Energy cost of absorption and metabolism in the ruminant gastrointestinal tract and liver: a review. J Anim Sci 1990;68:2997–3010.
2. Gill M, France J, Summers M, et al. Simulation of the energy costs associated with protein turnover and Na+,K+-transport in growing lambs. J Nutr 1989;119: 1287–99.
3. Johnson DE, Johnson KA, Baldwin RL. Changes in liver and gastrointestinal tract energy demands in response to physiological workload in ruminants. J Nutr 1990; 120:649–55.
4. Freetly HC, Ferrell CL, Jenkins TG, et al. Visceral oxygen consumption during chronic feed restriction and realimentation in sheep. J Anim Sci 1995;73:843–52.
5. Ferrell CL, Koong LJ, Nienaber JA. Effect of previous nutrition on body composition and maintenance energy costs of growing lambs. Br J Nutr 1986;56: 595–605.
6. Burrin DG, Ferrell CL, Eisemann JH, et al. Effect of level of nutrition on splanchnic blood flow and oxygen consumption in sheep. Br J Nutr 1989;62:23–34.
7. Burrin DG, Britton RA, Ferrell CL, et al. Level of nutrition and visceral organ size and metabolic activity in sheep. Br J Nutr 1990;64:439–48.
8. Wester TJ, Britton RA, Klopfenstein TJ, et al. Differential effects of plane of protein or energy nutrition on visceral organs and hormones in lambs. J Anim Sci 1995; 73:1674–88.
9. McLeod KR, Baldwin RL, VI. Effects of diet forage-to-concentrate ratio and metabolizable energy intake on visceral organ growth and in vitro oxidative capacity of gut tissues in sheep. J Anim Sci 2000;78:760–70.
10. Baldwin RL VI, McLeod KR. Effects of diet forage-to-concentrate ratio and metabolizable energy intake on isolated rumen epithelial cell substrate metabolism in vitro. J Anim Sci 2000;78:771–83.
11. Galfi P, Neogrady S, Sakata T. Effects of volatile fatty acids on the epithelial cell proliferation of the digestive tract and its hormonal mediation. In: Tsuda T, Sasaki Y, Kawashima R, editors. Physiological aspects of digestion and

metabolism in ruminants: proceedings of the Seventh International Symposium on Ruminant Physiology. San Diego (CA): Academic Press; 1991. p. 49–59.

12. Stevens CE. Fatty acid transport through the rumen epithelium. In: Phillipson AT, editor. Physiology of digestion and metabolism in the ruminant. Newcastle upon Tyne (United Kingdom): Oriel Press; 1969. p. 101–12.

13. Steven DH, Marshall AB. Organization of the rumen epithelium. In: Phillipson AT, editor. Physiology of digestion and metabolism in the ruminant. Newcastle upon Tyne (United Kingdom): Oriel Press; 1969. p. 80–100.

14. Steele MA, Penner GB, Chaucheyras-Durand F, et al. Development and physiology of the rumen and the lower gut: targets for improving gut health. J Dairy Sci 2016;99:4955–66.

15. Baldwin RL, Jesse BW. A technical note concerning the isolation and characterization of sheep rumen epithelial cells. J Anim Sci 1991;69:3603–9.

16. Tamate H, Kikuchi T, Sakata T. Ultrastructural changes in the ruminal epithelium after fasting and subsequent refeeding in the sheep. Tohoku J Agr Res 1974; 25:142.

17. Gaebel G, Martens H, Suendermann M, et al. The effect of diet, intraruminal pH and osmolarity on sodium, chloride and magnesium absorption from the temporarily isolated and washed reticulo-rumen of sheep. Quart J Exp Physiol 1987;72: 501–11.

18. Sakata T, Tamate H. Effect of intermittent feeding on the mitotic index and the ultrastructure of basal cells of the ruminal epithelium in the sheep. Tohoku J Agr Res 1974;25:156.

19. Stobo IJF, Roy JHB, Gaston HJ. Rumen development in the calf. Br J Nutr 1966; 20:171–88.

20. Harfoot CG. Anatomy, physiology and microbiology of the ruminant digestive tract. Prog Lipid Res 1978;17:1–19.

21. Church DC. Digestive physiology and nutrition of ruminants, vol. 1. Corvallis (OR): DC Church Publishing; 1975.

22. Annison EF, Hill KJ, Lewis D. Studies on the portal blood of sheep. 2. Absorption of volatile fatty acids from the rumen of the sheep. Biochem J 1957;66:592–9.

23. Kristensen NB, Huntington GB, Harmon DL. Splanchnic carbohydrate and energy metabolism in growing ruminants. In: Burrin DG, Mersman HJ, editors. Biology of growing animals series. Biology of metabolism in growing animals. Boston: Elsevier; 2005. p. 405–32.

24. Nocek JE, Herbein JH, Polan CE. Influence of ration physical form, ruminal degradable nitrogen and age on rumen epithelial propionate and acetate transport and some enzymatic activities. J Nutr 1980;110:2355–66.

25. Goosen PCM. Metabolism in rumen epithelium. Oxidation of substrates and formation of ketone bodies by pieces of rumen epithelium. Z Tierphysiol Tierernahr Futtermittelkd 1976;37:14–25.

26. Weekes TEC. The in vitro metabolism of propionate and glucose by the rumen epithelium. Comp Biochem Physiol 1974;49B:393–406.

27. Weigand E, Young JW, McGilliard AD. Volatile fatty acid metabolism by rumen mucosa from cattle fed hay or grain. J Dairy Sci 1975;58:1294–300.

28. Emmanuel B. Further metabolic studies in the rumen epithelium of camel (*Camelus dromedarius*) and sheep (*Ovis aries*). Comp Biochem Physiol 1981;68b: 155–8.

29. Baldwin RL VI, Jesse BW. Propionate modulation of ruminal ketogenesis. J Anim Sci 1996;74:1694–700.

30. Heitmann RN, Dawes DJ, Sensenig SC. Hepatic ketogenesis and peripheral ketone body utilization in the ruminant. J Nutr 1987;117:1174–80.

31. Beck U, Emmanuel B, Giesecke D. The ketogenic effect of glucose in rumen epithelium of ovine (*Ovis aries*) and bovine (*Bos taurus*) origin. Comp Biochem Physiol 1984;77B:517–21.

32. Leighton B, Nicholas AR, Pogson CI. The pathway of ketogenesis in rumen epithelium of the sheep. Biochem J 1983;216:769–72.

33. Bush RS, Milligan LP. Enzymes of ketogenesis in bovine rumen epithelium. Can J Anim Sci 1971a;51:129–33.

34. Warner RG, Flatt WP, Loosli JK. Dietary factors influencing the development of the ruminant stomach. Agric Food Chem 1956;4:788–801.

35. Gilliland RL, Bush LJ, Friend JD. Relation of ration composition to rumen development in early-weaned dairy calves with observations on ruminal parakeratosis. J Dairy Sci 1962;45:1211–7.

36. Giesecke D, Beck U, Wiesmayer S, et al. The effect of rumen epithelial development on metabolic activities and ketogenesis by the tissue *in vitro*. Comp Biochem Physiol 1979;62B:459–63.

37. Hamada T, Maeda S, Kameoka K. Factors influencing growth of rumen, liver, and other organs in kids weaned from milk replacers to solid foods. J Dairy Sci 1976;59:1110–8.

38. Sander EG, Warner RG, Harrison HN, et al. The stimulatory effect of sodium butyrate and sodium propionate on the development of rumen mucosa in the young calf. J Dairy Sci 1959;42:1600–5.

39. Tamate H, McGilliard AD, Jacobson NL, et al. Effect of various dietaries on the anatomical development of the stomach in the calf. J Dairy Sci 1962;45:408–20.

40. Lane MA, Jesse BW. Effect of volatile fatty acid infusion on development of the rumen epithelium in neonatal sheep. J Dairy Sci 1997;80:740–6.

41. Connor EE, Baldwin RL, Li C, et al. Gene expression in bovine rumen epithelium during weaning identifies molecular regulators of rumen development and growth. Funct Integr Genomics 2013;13:133–42.

42. Baldwin RL, Jesse BW. Developmental changes in glucose and butyrate metabolism by isolated sheep ruminal cells. J Nutr 1992;122:1149–53.

43. Smith RH. The development and function of the rumen in milk-fed calves. II. Effect of wood shavings in the diet. J Agric Sci 1961;56:105–13.

44. Orskov ER, Benzie D, Kay RNB. The effects of feeding procedure on closure of the oesophageal groove in young sheep. Br J Nutr 1970;24:785–94.

45. Rickard MD, Ternouth JH. The effect of the increased dietary volatile fatty acids on the morphological and physiological development of lambs with particular reference to the rumen. J Agric Sci 1965;65:371–82.

46. Sakata T, Tamate H. Effect of intraruminal injection of n-sodium butyrate on the mitotic indices in sheep ruminal epithelium. Tohoku J Agr Res 1976;27:133–5.

47. Sakata T, Tamate H. Effect of n-butyrate administration rate on the epithelial cell proliferation in adult sheep rumen: a preliminary report. Tohoku J Agr Res 1976;27:136–8.

48. Sakata T, Tamate H. Rumen epithelial cell proliferation accelerated by rapid increase in intraruminal butyrate. J Dairy Sci 1978;61:1109–13.

49. Sakata T, Tamate H. Rumen epithelium cell proliferation accelerated by propionate and acetate. J Dairy Sci 1979;62:49–52.

50. Gálfi P, Veresegyházy T, Neogrády S, et al. Effect of sodium n-butyrate on primary ruminal epithelial cell culture. Zender Veter Med 1981;28:259–61.

51. Baldwin RL VI. The proliferative actions of insulin, insulin-like growth factor-I, epidermal growth factor, butyrate and propionate on ruminal epithelial cells in vitro. Small Ruminant Res 1999;32:261–8.
52. Sakata T, Hikosaka K, Shiomura Y, et al. Stimulatory effect of insulin on ruminal epithelium cell mitosis in adult sheep. Br J Nutr 1980;44:325–31.
53. Galfi P, Neogrady S. Epithelial and non-epithelial cell- and tissue culture from the rumen mucosa. Asian-Australas J Anim Sci 1989;2:143–9.
54. White RG, Leng RA. Glucose metabolism in feeding and postabsorptive lambs and mature sheep. Comp Biochem Physiol 1980;67A:223–9.
55. Lane MA, Baldwin RL VI, Jesse BW. Sheep rumen metabolic development in response to different dietary treatments. J Anim Sci 2000;78:1990–6.
56. Lane MA, Baldwin RL, Jesse BW. Developmental changes in ketogenic enzyme gene expression during sheep rumen development. J Anim Sci 2002;80: 1538–44.
57. Baldwin RL VI, Wu S, Li W, et al. Quantification of transcriptome responses of the rumen epithelium to butyrate infusion using RNA-seq technology. Gene Regul Syst Bio 2012;6:67–80.
58. Steele MA, Vandervoort G, AlZahal O, et al. Rumen epithelial adaptation to high-grain diets involves the coordinated regulation of genes involved in cholesterol homeostasis. Physiol Genomics 2011;43:308–16.
59. Kinoshita M, Suzuki Y, Saito Y. Butyrate reduces colonic paracellular permeability by enhancing PPARγ activation. Biochem Biophys Res Commun 2002;293: 827–31.
60. Penner GB, Steele MA, Aschenbach JR, et al. Ruminant nutrition symposium: molecular adaptation of ruminal epithelia to highly fermentable diets. J Anim Sci 2011;89:1108–19.
61. Naeem A, Drackley JK, Stamey J, et al. Role of metabolic and cellular proliferation genes in ruminal development in response to enhanced plane of nutrition in neonatal Holstein calves. J Dairy Sci 2012;95:1807–20.

Diagnostic Approach to Forestomach Diseases

Dusty W. Nagy, DVM, MS, PhD

KEYWORDS

- Forestomach diseases • Rumen fluid analysis • Ultrasonography • Radiography

KEY POINTS

- A complete physical examination is the core to approaching disease of the ruminant forestomach.
- Rumen fluid analysis will help to determine the heath of the rumen and aid in diagnosis of fermentative disorders.
- Ultrasound is a useful tool in identifying motility disorders of the forestomach; however, it lacks some specificity in identification of the exact disease process. It performs best in cases of traumatic reticuloperitonitis.

 Video content accompanies this article at http://www.vetfood.theclinics.com.

INTRODUCTION

Diseases of the gastrointestinal system are commonly seen by the ruminant practitioner. Forestomach disease in the ruminant animal can be divided into primary and secondary causes. Primary diseases of the forestomach are caused by disruptions in the ruminal wall and contraction cycle or by a disruption in the normal flora and fermentation processes of the rumen. Secondary disease of the reticulorumen is caused by abnormalities in rumen contraction and/or fermentation secondary to other systemic illnesses. It is important to recognize that rumen function is complex and that the contraction cycle and fermentation are deeply inter-related. As such, diseases of contraction will eventually result in fermentation abnormalities and vice versa. This article will focus on the diagnostic approach to this general group of diseases.

PATIENT HISTORY

As with all disease investigations, a good history will help build a reasonable list of differential diagnoses. Routine information such as signalment, chief complaint, initial

The author has nothing to disclose.
Department of Veterinary Medicine and Surgery, University of Missouri, College of Veterinary Medicine, 900 East Campus Drive, Columbia, MO 65211, USA
E-mail address: nagyd@missouri.edu

clinical signs, duration of signs, onset (gradual or sudden), and progression (slow or rapid) may all be helpful. In addition, detailed information regarding the diet (type, formulation, duration of feeding, recent or historical changes in components, amount fed, or amount consumed) should be obtained. The mixed diet and potentially components should be visualized for fiber length, moisture, odor, and obvious abnormalities such as mold, spoilage, and contamination.

PHYSICAL EXAMINATION

Understanding the location, structure, and function of the forestomach is critical to the examination. The rumen occupies the left side of the abdomen immediately distal to the diaphragm to the pelvic inlet. The cardia can be found slightly above the middle of the seventh intercostal space (ICS) or eighth rib, while the dorsal blind sac of the rumen will be just cranial to the pelvis when the rumen is full.[1] The ventral sac will cross slightly over midline in the normal animal. As it progresses caudally, the ventral sac may come close to the right body wall. The reticulum is located to the left of midline cranioventrally at the level of ribs 6 to 8 immediately caudal to the diaphragm. The omasum lies to the right of midline adjacent to the rumen and reticulum and to the left of the liver under ribs 8 to 11. Evaluation of the forestomach should include an assessment of contraction rate and strength, as well as abdominal and rumen contour, and an assessment of rumen fill.

Rumenoreticular motility incorporates 3 contraction patterns responsible for mixing, eructation, and rumination.[2,3] Primary contractions are responsible for mixing of ingesta and maintaining the normal stratification of rumen contents. These start as a biphasic reticular contraction that moves ingesta dorsocaudally into the rumen. Contraction of the dorsal rumen sac while the ventral sac relaxes will force ingesta into the ventral rumen. After this, a wavelike contraction involving the caudoventral sac, caudodorsal sac, and ventral sac will move ingesta into the reticulum and cranial rumen. Particles of 2 to 4 mm or smaller will pass through the reticulo-omasal orifice at the next reticular contraction. Primary contractions occur at a rate of 50 to 100 contractions per hour.

Secondary contractions will allow for eructation of excessive gas in response to stimulation of tension receptors within the rumen. Contraction of the dorsal and caudodorsal rumen sacs will force gas cranially. At the same time, contraction of the rumenoreticular fold will inhibit ingesta from moving to the cardia. Receptors at the cardia detect the gas and open, allowing for the eructation of gas. Secondary contractions occur every 2 minutes and can be confirmed by the eructation of gas.

The presence of coarse feed in the rumen can be sensed by receptors in the reticulum, rumenoreticular fold, ruminal pillars, and esophageal groove. This stimulates the vagus nerve, causing an extrareticular contraction prior to the primary contraction cycle. During inspiration, the glottis closes, and the cardia opens, allowing a bolus of ingesta to enter the distal esophagus. This bolus is delivered to the mouth by reverse peristalsis. Rumination typically begins 30 minutes after eating and continues in 10- to 60-minute cycles. The total amount of time ruminating will depend greatly on feed type. The more course the feed, the more time cows will spend ruminating.

Physical examination of the omasum is rarely undertaken. The contractions are more regular than those of the rumenoreticulum.[1] The contractions are biphasic, with the first portion pushing ingesta into the laminae and squeezing out the fluid. The second phase is a whole-organ contraction that moves ingesta into the abomasum.

In the healthy cow, rumen contractions should be easily ausculted in the left paralumbar fossa at a rate of 2 to 3 contractions per 2 minutes. In most clinical settings, no attempts are made to auscult the reticulum independently of the rumen contraction cycle. If interested, reticular contractions can be heard as a tinkling sound with a stethoscope placed at the seventh ICS at the level of the costochondral junction.[3] If the examiner leans into the left paralumbar fossa with a fist is placed in the fossa, normal rumen contractions should have the strength to easily push the examiner away from the cow. The normal rumen should not ping or have sucussable fluid present. Severe cases of free gas bloat will increase the tension enough to generate a rumen ping. More commonly, the rumen will ping from the decreased fill associated with a rumen void. In these cases, a ping can be found on the left along the dorsal abdominal wall and off the transverse processes. Despite having a large fluid phase to the ingesta present in the rumen, the normal tone and fiber mat will prevent the auscultation of sucussable fluid. Diseases that cause significant disruption of the fiber mat and decreased rumen tone, such as acute carbohydrate overload, may result in the presence of sucussable fluid.

If the rumen is palpated externally through the left body wall, a change in the consistency and resistance to palpation can be noted. The gas cap can be felt high in the left paralumbar fossa. The fiber mat is firm and somewhat indentable. As palpation progresses more ventrally, the indentable mat will become firm and poorly pliable as the fluid phase is reached. The exact location of the junction between fiber mat and fluid phase is difficult to determine. On rectal examination, the dorsal aspect of the rumen can be palpated. The gas cap and fiber mat can be palpated. The normal fiber mat will indent when pushed on and slowly return to form similar to compressing bread dough. The left longitundinal groove is palpated as an indentation where the dorsal and ventral rumen sacs meet. The dorsal portion of the ventral sac is also typically palpable. Enlargement of the ventral sac of the rumen with fluid, froth, or ingesta is easily palpable per rectum as the ventral sac distends. However, the exact nature of the ingesta within the distended viscus is difficult to determine.

Attention to abdominal contour will also yield information regarding the origin of disease in the patient. Diseases that impair outflow from the rumen, whether it is gas from inappropriate eructation or ingesta from impaired aboral flow, will cause observable distention of the abdomen. Gas build up from failure to eructate will cause an increase in the size of the rumen gas cap. This will cause distention high on the left side of the cow. In severe cases, it may billow out from under the transverse processes and course further dorsally. If ingesta fails to leave the rumen appropriately, distention will begin low on the right; as the ventral sac fills and distends, it will cross over to the right side of the abdomen. If normal aboral flow is not reestablished, the rumen will continue to fill, and distention will be notable low on the left and right and progress toward filling more dorsally on the right in the most severe cases.

DIAGNOSTIC TESTING
Rumen Fluid Analysis

The method of rumen fluid collection is often debated.[4–6] The major drawback to sample collection by orogastric intubation is the potential for sample contamination with saliva. This may affect the measurement of multiple analytes, but none as clinically relevant as pH. As monitoring rumen pH becomes more common as a herd survey tool for detecting subacute rumen acidosis, the integrity of this measurement becomes more important and often favors rumenocentesis.[4,5,7] The major drawbacks to rumenocentesis are the need for a surgical preparation and the potential for abdominal contamination and resulting risk of peritonitis.[4] While a strong case can be made for collecting rumen fluid samples by rumenocentesis for pH evaluation in investigations for subacute rumen acidosis, orogastric intubation should be more than adequate for rumen fluid collection for routine analysis in sick individual cows.

The ideal site for collection of rumen fluid for pH evaluation is the ventral rumen sac, as salvia should be minimally present, and rumen fluid should be abundant.[7,8] Studies looking at analytes such as volatile fatty acids, ammonia, and others have suggested that sampling in the central rumen is most appropriate.[9] Traditional stomach tubes are often difficult to pass through the fibrous mat layer to reach the fluid phase. This can be overcome by use of a weighted stomach tube that has fenestrated steel at the end. This will allow for the tube to more easily sink below the fiber mat. Minimum requirements to ensure appropriate tube placement and capacity to retrieve fluid are a tube that is 2.3 m long and 9 mm in diameter. Commercial tubes (Dirksen, Selekt Rumen Fluid Collector) are available that are designed to pass beyond the fiber mat and allow for collection of fluid from the ventral rumen. These tubes, when used according to directions, have been found to accurately measure rumen pH.[10] The influence of site of collection on common field tests like new methylene blue reduction, protozoal count and motility, and bacterial populations have not been evaluated.

Rumenocentesis can be achieved by restraining the cow in a chute or stanchion. Sedation can be used, but application of a tail jack is often sufficient restraint. The location for puncture on the left side is 15 to 20 cm posterior to the last rib on a horizontal line even with the dorsal aspect of the patella.[4] The area should be clipped and surgically prepped. A 4 inch to -5 inch, 16-gauge needle is then passed through the skin into the rumen. Minimal pressure should be applied to aspirate fluid, as negative pressure will release CO_2 and raise the pH.[5,11] If the needled becomes clogged by ingesta, a small amount of fluid can be pushed back in to free the needle tip. Typically 3 to 15 mL of fluid are obtained.

Although controversy remains over the methodology of collection, it is clear that both rumenocentesis and orogastric intubation can both be used to collect samples for analysis when the described methods are followed. The required sample size for the tests to be run should be considered when choosing a method, as rumenocentesis will only reliably yield small volumes that are inadequate for a complete analysis.

Various parameters, including color, consistency, smell, protozoal composition and activity, bacterial composition, pH, methylene blue reduction, and sedimentation rate, have all been utilized to provide information regarding rumen health.[8,12] Rumen chloride concentration is also measured, but is primarily used to assess for reflux associated with abomasal or proximal intestinal abnormalities. Color, consistency, and smell can all be evaluated at the time of collection. Normal findings will vary depending on feed type (**Table 1**), while abnormalities may lead toward a specific diagnosis (**Table 2**).[8,12]

The pH should be assessed immediately after collection. Exposure to air may artificially increase pH, while ongoing fermentation may artificially decrease pH.[4,5] In

Table 1
Parameters for color, smell, viscosity, and methylene blue reduction in normal animals based on diet

Diet	Color	Smell	Viscosity	pH	Methylene Blue Reduction (min)
Forage	Green	Aromatic	Slightly viscous	6.0–7.2	6–8
Silage/grain	Yellow-brown	Aromatic	Slightly viscous	5.5–6.5	3–6
Mixed forage/grain	Green-brown	Aromatic	Slightly viscous		<3–4

Table 2
Parameters for color, smell, viscosity, and pH in selected disease states

Condition	Color	Smell	Viscosity	pH	Methylene Blue Reduction
Anorexia Indigestion		Stale but not foul	Watery	7.0–7.5	
Prolonged atony with putrefaction	Dark brown-black	Rancid	Watery	7.0–7.5	
Ruminal acidosis	Gray	Sour, acidic	Watery	<5.5 SARA <5.0 acute	
Urea toxicity		Ammonia		>8.0	
Abomasal reflux	Dark brown	Bitter almonds; burned popcorn		<5.5	

addition, saliva contamination during collection may falsely elevate the pH on samples collected by orogastric intubation.[4,5] The time between eating and sample collection will also alter rumen pH and should be taken into account when interpreting the results. pH is at its lowest approximately 3 to 5 hours after feeding. It is important to recognize that rumen pH may shift relatively quickly, especially in cases of acute grain overload (6–24 hours), so the measured pH may not always reflect the disease process. In these cases, microbial population evaluation may be helpful in determining the cause of disease.

The redox potential of the rumen is primarily maintained by the microbial population of the rumen and can be measured by using a methylene blue reduction test.[8] To perform the test, 0.5 mL of 0.03% methylene blue should be mixed with 10 mL of fresh rumen fluid, which may be strained if needed to remove particulate matter. The time for the sample to clear the blue color to a matched control should be measured (**Fig. 1**). At the end of the test, a blue ring may be left at the top of the sample. The higher the microbial activity, the shorter the time for the sample to clear (see **Table 1**). Prolonged reduction over 10 minutes is indicative of inactive microflora.

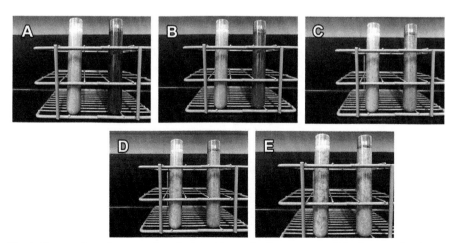

Fig. 1. Progression of a normal methylene blue reduction test over 3.5 minutes. The ring at the top of the tube in the last image is considered normal at the end of the test.

Sedimentation activity time is a qualitative measurement of microbial activity.[8,13] It will not help to diagnose an exact malady, but will give an idea of microbial activity. This should be performed on fresh rumen fluid immediately after collection. For this test, a sample of rumen fluid is placed in a cylinder and placed where it can sit undisturbed. The start time should be recorded. Small particulate matter will settle, while larger particles will float to the surface due to microbial gas production (**Fig. 2**). Typical flotation time takes 4 to 8 minutes and is most active in forage-fed animals. Animals on high carbohydrate and pelleted diets will have rapid sedimentation with minimal particle flotation. Frothy bloat will have particles suspended within the fluid for extended periods of time and may not show any flotation.

The presence and activity of the microbial population should also be evaluated.[8,12,14] Protozoa can be evaluated by placing a drop of fresh, warm rumen fluid on a slide. Large numbers of motile protozoa of varying sizes should be present (Video 1). A drop of Giemsa or Wright stain can be added to enhance contrast (Video 2). Lugols iodine can be used to stop motility and allow counting of protozoa if desired, but counting protozoal numbers are generally not necessary for adequate interpretation. Protozoal numbers will be decreased with most disease processes that affect the rumen. Large and medium protozoa are most susceptible to ruminal environmental change and will die first, leaving the more active small protozoa behind. Similarly, as protozoa repopulate after an insult, small organisms will return first, followed by the medium then large. Lack of protozoa suggests that rumen pH has dropped below 5 in the recent past, killing all ciliates present in the rumen. In addition to protozoa, an assessment of the bacterial population can be made by Gram staining the fluid.[8,14] In the normal rumen, there is a predominance of Gram-negative bacteria. In cases of acute carbohydrate overload the bacterial population changes primarily Gram positive.

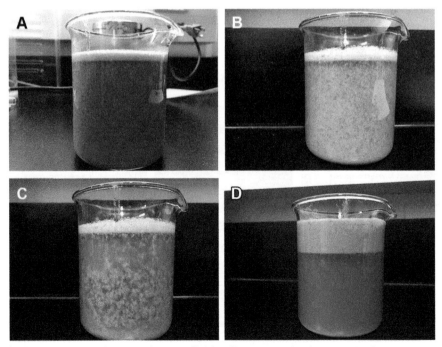

Fig. 2. Progression of a normal rumen fluid sediment examination over 4 minutes.

Rumen chloride concentration is not routinely completed with rumen fluid analysis and is typically reserved for conditions in which reflux of abomasal contents into the rumen is suspected. Normal rumen chloride in the cow is 15 to 30 mEq/L.[12] In diseases that cause partial or complete abomasal outflow obstruction or generalized ileus, this value will be elevated.

Radiography

Radiography has limited diagnostic capacity in the investigation of forestomach disease. Capturing static images in a motile, dynamic environment limits the ability of radiographs to evaluate contractility and may also allow for misinterpretation of wall conformation based on the presence of contractions. The size of the animal also limits the capacity to take orthogonal views. Access to only lateral images will limit the capacity to triangulate and evaluate objects and organs in 2dimensions.

The utility of radiography lies mostly in the investigation of suspected cases of traumatic reticuloperitonitis. Reticular films can be obtained in the standing or dorsally recumbent animal.[15–17] The width of the thorax at the eighth rib between the elbow and shoulder should be measured for machine settings. The cassette should be placed 5 to 15 cm from the left thoracic wall parallel to the animal. The eighth rib should be aligned with the middle of the cassette, and the ventral border of the cassette should be parallel to the ventral abdominal wall.

One study evaluating the utility of radiographs in the diagnosis of traumatic reticuloperitonitis found the sensitivity of radiographs to be between 64% and 96% and specificity to be between 19% and 80% depending on the radiographic parameter observed.[17] Higher sensitivities were associated with reticular content (presence of foreign body). Higher specificities were associated with reticular contour, the presence of gas or gas-fluid interfaces within the reticulum, and abnormal findings within the cranioventral abdomen (soft tissue mass, gas, or gas fluid interfaces). Contour of the reticular wall and abnormal findings in the cranioventral abdomen had the highest positive predictive values at 92% and 96%, respectively.

When compared with ultrasonography in the diagnosis of traumatic reticuloperitonitis, the 2 diagnostic modalities are somewhat complementary. Radiography was better suited to find foreign bodies, whereas ultrasound was better able to find abscesses, peritonitis, and chronic adhesions associated with traumatic reticuloperitonitis.[17–19] In addition, ultrasonography has some utility in follow-up during treatment for cases of traumatic reticuloperitonitis.[20]

Ultrasound

Ultrasound is uniquely suited for examination of the ruminant forestomach, as it allows for assessment of both structure and function. In addition to organ placement and contour, ultrasound allows for the identification of soft tissue structures such as abscesses and fibrin or fibrinous deposits that are more difficult to identify on radiographs. The frequency and amplitude of organ contractions can also be evaluated. It is important to recognize that the size of cattle limits visualization of some organs. In addition, not all parts can be visualized all of the time, even in the normal animal. The utility of ultrasound is proportional to experience of the operator and the quality of the machine. This is a skill that takes practice in obtaining adequate images as well as interpreting what is found. Ultrasound quality cannot be overlooked, as lower quality machines do not always have the resolution to allow differentiation of closely related objects. Publications are available that detail image acquisition and interpretation of the gastrointestinal system of normal and some abnormal cattle.[21–25]

Several studies have investigated the use of ultrasound in evaluating the forestomach of cattle. Fewer have attempted to set forth normal parameters in health and disease. Ultrasound of the rumen in dairy cattle has been investigated.[23] The dorsal and ventral ruminal sacs and the left longitudinal groove are reliably imaged in cows. The dorsal sac of the rumen can be found from the tenth ICS to caudal flank, while the ventral sac of the rumen can be found from the eleventh ICS to the caudal flank. In some normal cattle, they can be identified more cranially, but detection at these locations is less reliable. The height of both sacs is variable throughout the left side, often due to superimposition of other organs. The maximum height of the dorsal sac was greatest at the caudal flank, with a mean of 40.3 cm and of the ventral sac was greatest at the twelfth ICS, with a mean of 62.6 cm. Ruminal wall thickness is fairly uniform at 0.3 cm. Although it is possible to determine the junction between dorsal rumen gas cap and the fiber mat, the differentiation between fiber mat and fluid phase is not as easily distinguished.

Ultrasonographic assessment of reticular motility has also been evaluated in cows at rest, while eating and during periods of stress.[24] The normal biphasic reticular contraction can be seen ultrasonographically during all of these activities. Contraction rates on average were 3.6 contractions every 3 minutes while at rest, 4.6 contractions every 3 minutes while eating, 3.2 contractions every 3 minutes while ruminating, and 3.1 contractions per 3 minutes while stressed. Contraction duration was between 2.4 and 3.0 seconds for the first reticular contraction and between 4.0 and 4.3 seconds for the second depending on activity of the cow. The amplitude ranged from 7.9 to 8.7 cm for the first contraction and 9.9 to 11.2 cm for the second. The additional reticular contraction that occurs while ruminating lasted a mean of 3.2 seconds, with an amplitude of 8 cm. Of all the data collected in the study, only the number of contractions, the duration of the first reticular contraction, and the time between the biphasic contractions were significantly different depending on activity of the cow.

A study that evaluated reticular contractions in cattle with vagal indigestion found no differences in reticular position, contour, size, contraction rate, or amplitude.[26] Differences were present in reticular contraction rate between cows with failure of omasal transport (4.6 contractions every 3 minutes) and pyloric outflow failure (3.6 contractions every 3 minutes).[26] It is important to recognize that although significantly different, the range of the data was wide, with cows in both groups having reticular atony, and some cows having up to 8 contractions every 3 minutes. The means of the contraction rates in the cattle with vagal indigestion also fell within the published normal range for some activity levels.

The normal omasum can be found on the right under ribs 8 to 11. Using a 3.5 MHz transducer, it can be identified most reliably at the eighth and ninth ICS.[25] At the level of the eighth ICS, the upper limit can be found approximately 56.1 cm ventral to the dorsal midline and the lower limit approximately 99.3 cm ventral to the dorsal midline at a depth ranging from 4 to 10 cm depending on location. The ninth ICS the upper limit can be found approximately 51.3 cm ventral to the dorsal midline and the lower limit approximately 108.2 cm ventral to the dorsal midline at a depth of 5 to 12 cm depending on location. In normal cattle, contractions are not noted ultrasonographically. In addition, only the attachments of the lamellae can be seen. In animals with nonomasal gastrointestinal disease, the omasum may be found in an alternate location, and in some, the lamellae can be seen as thin echogenic lines, suggesting an increased fluid content of the omasum.[26,27] In animals with left displacement of the abomasum, the omasum was shifted cranial and ventral. With abomasal volvulus, it was shifted ventrally. With ileus, the ventral border was shifted dorsally, with minimal alteration to the dorsal border. In animals with reticulo-omasal stenosis, the omasum was shifted dorsally, and contractions are more readily visualized.

Overall, the approach to diagnosis of forestomach disorders is a multifaceted process rooted in the physical examination with fine tuning through the use of several tools available to the veterinarian. The history and examination should help dictate which of the tools or combinations of tools (rumen fluid analysis, radiography, ultrasonography) should be pursued to best identify the problem and plan of action for the individual patient.

SUPPLEMENTARY DATA

Supplementary data related to this article can be found online at http://dx.doi.org/10.1016/j.cvfa.2017.06.002.

REFERENCES

1. Dyce KM, Sack WO, Wensing CJG. The abdomen of ruminants. In: Textbook of veterinary anatomy. 3rd edition. Philadelphia: Elsevier Science (USA); 1987. p. 666–90.
2. Kay RNB. Rumen function and physiology. Vet Rec 1983;113:6–9.
3. Leek BF. Clinical diseases of the rumen: a physiologist's review. Vet Rec 1983; 113:10–4.
4. Nordlund KV, Garrett EF. Rumenocentesis: a technique for the diagnosis of subacute rumen acidosis in dairy herds. Bov Pract 1994;28:109–12.
5. Garrett EF, Pereira MN, Nordlund KV, et al. Diagnostic methods for detecting subacute ruminal acidosis in dairy cattle. J Dairy Sci 1999;82:1170–8.
6. Keefe GP, Ogilvie TH. Comparison of oro-rumenal probe and rumenocentesis for prediction of rumen pH in dairy cattle. Proc Am Assoc Bovine Prac 1997;30: 168–9.
7. Duffield T, Plaizier JC, Fairfield A, et al. Comparison of techniques for measurement of pH in lactating dairy cows. J Dairy Sci 2004;87:59–66.
8. Dirksen G, Smith MC. Acquisition and analysis of bovine rumen fluid. Bov Pract 1987;22:108–16.
9. Shen JS, Chai Z, Song LJ, et al. Insertion depth of oral stomach tubes may affect the fermentation parameters of ruminal fluid collected in dairy cows. J Dairy Sci 2012;95:5978–84.
10. Steiner S, Neidl A, Linhart N, et al. Randomised prospective study compares efficacy of five different stomach tubes for rumen fluid sampling in dairy cows. Vet Rec 2015;176(2):50.
11. Smith VR. In Vivo studies of hydrogen ion concentrations in the rumen of the dairy cow. J Dairy Sci 1941;24:659–65.
12. Radostits OM, Gay CC, Hinchcliff KW, et al, editors. Examination of rumen fluid. Veterinary medicine. A textbook of the diseases of cattle, horses, sheep, pigs, and goats. 10th edition. Philadelphia: Saunders Elsevier; 2007. p. 304–5.
13. Nichols RE, Penn KE. Simple methods for the detection of unfavorable changes in ruminal ingesta. J Am Vet Med Assoc 1958;133:275–7.
14. Pounden WD. Rumen sampling: a diagnostic aid. Vet Med 1954;49:221–5, 228.
15. Ducharme NG, Dill SG, Rendano VT. Reticulography of the cow in dorsal recumbency: an aid in the diagnosis and treatment of traumatic reticuloperitonitis. J Am Vet Med Assoc 1983;182(6):585–8.

16. Fubini SL, Yeager AE, Mohammed HO, et al. Accuracy of radiography of the reticulum for predicting surgical findings in adult dairy cattle with traumatic reticuloperitonitis: 123 cases (1981-1987). J Am Vet Med Assoc 1990;197(8):1060–4.

17. Braun U, Flückiger M, Nägeli F. Radiograpgy as an aid in the diagnosis of traumatic reticuloperitonitis in cattle. Vet Rec 1993;132:103–9.

18. Braun U, Götz M, Marimier O. Ultrasonographic findings in cows with traumatic reticuloperitonitis. Vet Rec 1993;133:416–22.

19. Braun U, Flückiger M, Götz M. Comparison of ultrasonographic and radiographic findings in cows with traumatic reticuloperitonitis. Vet Rec 1994;135:470–8.

20. Braun U, Iselin U, Lischer C, et al. Ultrasonographic findings in five cows before and after treatment of reticular abscesses. Vet Rec 1998;142:184–9.

21. Braun U. Ultrasonography of the gastrointestinal tract in cattle. Vet Clin North Am Food Anim Pract 2009;25:567–90.

22. Braun U. Ultrasonography in gastrointestinal disease in cattle. Vet J 2003;166: 112–24.

23. Braun U, Schweizer A, Trösch L. Ultrasonography of the rumen in dairy cows. BMC Vet Res 2013;9:44.

24. Braun U, Rauch S. Ultrasonographic evaluation of reticular motility during rest, eating, rumination, and stress in 30 healthy cows. Vet Rec 2008;163:571–4.

25. Braun U, Blessing S. Ultrasonographic examination of the omasum in 30 healthy cows. Vet Rec 2006;159:812–5.

26. Braun U, Rauch S, Hässig M. Ultrasonographic evaluation of reticular motility in 144 cattle with vagal indigestion. Vet Rec 2009;164:11–3.

27. Braun U, Blessing S, Lejeune B, et al. Ultrasonography of the omasum in cows with various gastrointestinal diseases. Vet Rec 2007;160:865–9.

Diagnosis and Treatment of Clinical Rumen Acidosis

Emily Snyder, DVM, MFAM, Brent Credille, DVM, PhD*

KEYWORDS

- Acidosis • Rumenitis • Liver abscessation • Laminitis

KEY POINTS

- Although classically considered a disease of cattle fed in confinement, rumen acidosis is a common cause of morbidity and mortality in both small and large ruminant populations.
- Feeding and management practices that lead to consumption of large amounts of feed containing readily fermentable carbohydrates precipitate clinical disease.
- Sequelae to rumen acidosis include laminitis, rumen ulceration, liver abscessation, and thromboembolic respiratory disease, each of which can have a greater impact on animal health and well-being than the primary disease process.
- Treatment of the individual animal with rumen acidosis focuses on correction of volume deficits, supplementation of alkalinizing agents, restoration of a normal rumen microenvironment, and management of secondary complications.
- Prevention of rumen acidosis is centered on restricting access to feeds containing readily fermentable carbohydrates to which animals are not accustomed, gradually introducing feed containing concentrates over a period of weeks, and addressing management practices that promote aggressive eating behavior.

INTRODUCTION

Clinical rumen acidosis remains a major cause of morbidity and mortality in modern ruminant production systems. Survey data from feedlot cattle have revealed that approximately 4.4% of cattle placed on feed are diagnosed with digestive problems.[1] Similarly, it is estimated that anywhere from 14% to 42% of deaths in feedlot cattle are due to digestive disorders, making them the second leading cause of mortality in feedlots.[2,3] Acute rumen acidosis represents an economically important loss to the beef industry. It has been estimated that the average cost of treating cattle with acidosis

Disclosure Statement: The authors have nothing to disclose.
Food Animal Health and Management Program, Department of Population Health, University of Georgia College of Veterinary Medicine, Veterinary Medical Center, 2200 College Station Road, Athens, GA 30602, USA
* Corresponding author.
E-mail address: bc24@uga.edu

Vet Clin Food Anim 33 (2017) 451–461
http://dx.doi.org/10.1016/j.cvfa.2017.06.003
0749-0720/17/© 2017 Elsevier Inc. All rights reserved.

averages $10/head and, with an estimated 10.7 million cattle on feed as of December 1, 2016, this would translate to about $4.6 million in treatment costs alone.[4]

Although commonly viewed as a disease of cattle on high-concentrate rations, rumen acidosis has also been reported in sheep, goats, and New World camelids. Although few data are available evaluating the true incidence and impact of acidosis in these populations, it is thought that the disease occurs less frequently because of a combination of factors that include differences in behavior, feeding practices, and forestomach physiology. Nevertheless, clinical rumen acidosis can be responsible for considerable morbidity and mortality in some small ruminant populations, making recognition of the disease important for any practitioner.

This text reviews available data regarding the pathophysiology, clinical signs, diagnosis, treatment, and prevention of clinical rumen acidosis in cattle, sheep, goats, and New World camelids.

PATHOPHYSIOLOGY

Often viewed as the most dramatic form of the forestomach fermentative disorders, clinical ruminal acidosis occurs when excessive levels of organic acids accumulate in the rumen, resulting in a rumen fluid pH of less than 5.2.[2,5] A common scenario for the development of clinical rumen acidosis is the excessive consumption of rapidly fermentable carbohydrates by ruminants that are unadapted to a high-concentrate diet. As a result, clinical rumen acidosis is often seen in the early feeding period when newly received feedlot cattle, accustomed to a primarily forage-based diet, are introduced to a primarily concentrate-based ration and stepped up too rapidly.[2,3] Similar signs can also develop when concentrate-adapted ruminants are fed more concentrate than their ruminal microbial population can handle. This situation might occur following a feeding error, overprocessing of grain, changes in ration moisture, or when there is excessive competition for feed within an animal population.[5,6] Excessive feeding of rapidly fermentable carbohydrates, commonly referred to as "grain overload," is the classic scenario leading to clinical rumen acidosis. It is important to remember, however, that excess grain consumption is not essential to the development of the syndrome, because excess consumption of any rapidly fermentable carbohydrate (apples and other fruits, bakery waste products, incompletely fermented brewery products, and standing green corn) is capable of providing the necessary substrate for the development of clinical disease.[6] In fact, the authors have seen clinical rumen acidosis in mature does following consumption of excessive amounts of animal crackers given by the owners as treats.

Regardless of the initial inciting cause, the pathogenesis of clinical rumen acidosis is the same. Ruminal bacteria that digest starches and sugars proliferate and increase their rate of carbohydrate fermentation. In the normal animal, or in animals with mild clinical disease, rumen buffering capacity and volatile fatty acid (VFA) absorption match the rate of carbohydrate fermentation. In this scenario, the pH within the rumen will stay in a normal range between 5.6 and 6.9, with the higher pH range being more common in New World camelids.[5,7–9] However, when production of VFAs and lactate exceeds the rate of absorption, rumen pH will begin to drop. VFAs and lactate increase in concentration within the rumen fluid and are subsequently absorbed into the systemic circulation.[10] Although numerous microorganisms have been implicated in the development of disease, the primary bacterium thought to be associated with the progression of clinical signs is *Streptococcus bovis*. *S bovis*, because of its rapid rate of division, ability to produce more ATP per unit time, and tolerance of a pH <5.5, is the microorganism that sets the stage for acid production and worsening of symptoms.[7]

Nevertheless, *S bovis* is intolerant of a pH >4.5. As pH decreases, lactate production by *S bovis* decreases, and the growth of *S bovis* is slowed.[7] At this point, the *Lactobacilli* become the dominant microbes present in the rumen and further serve to depress ruminal pH.[2]

There are 2 chiral forms of lactate produced in the rumen: D and L. The L isomer is produced by both mammalian and microbial cells, whereas the D form is produced primarily by microbes.[5] The L-lactate is easily metabolized by mammalian cardiac and hepatic tissues. D-Lactate is not metabolized nearly as efficiently as L-lactate and accumulates in circulation.[5] For this reason, a more appropriate term for clinical rumen acidosis would be acute D-lactic acidosis.[11] Nevertheless, regardless of the form, lactate appears to be less readily absorbed across the rumen wall than are VFAs. Indeed, VFAs tend to be much weaker acids than either D- or L-lactate and serve as buffers in the rumen fluid. This phenomenon contributes to many of the VFAs existing in the nondissociated state, a factor that enhances their absorption into the systemic circulation.[12,13] Despite this, enough lactate is absorbed in the forestomach and more distal portions of the digestive tract to cause acidemia. Furthermore, many VFAs are transformed into lactate by the rumen wall to further add to the acid load in the bloodstream.[8,12] In addition, as rumen pH further declines, lactate starts to become the dominant organic acid present in significant amounts in the rumen. It is thought that the decrease in numbers of VFA-producing microbes and increased activity of pyruvate dehydrogenase in the acidic rumen environment promote the further accumulation of lactate.[5,7]

D- and L-Lactate are powerful corrosive agents that can cause severe damage to the rumen epithelium. In addition, lactate and VFAs are osmotically active. Increased rumen osmolarity decreases absorption of lactate and VFAs, creating a cycle that perpetuates buildup of these compounds and a continued drop in pH.[5,13] With the continued accumulation of these compounds and further increases in rumen fluid osmolarity, the rumen epithelium is further disrupted. Yeast and fungi that are resistant to highly acidic environments readily colonize the denuded sites and contribute to the development of mycotic rumenitis and omasitis. In addition, organisms such as *Fusobacterium necrophorum* are able to invade the bloodstream and spread to the liver. In fact, rumen acidosis is thought to be one of the inciting causes for the development of liver abscesses in ruminants. In addition to their effects on the rumen, the osmotic pressure of these agents causes systemic dehydration and hypovolemia by pulling fluid from the circulation into the rumen, resulting in a reduction in tissue perfusion.[5,14] The loss of circulating blood volume leads to cardiovascular collapse, reduced renal perfusion, and anuria. Reduced peripheral circulation also leads to anaerobic cellular metabolism and systemic acidosis.

In addition to lactate, there are many other compounds produced by rumen microbes that can be deleterious to multiple organ systems. Some of these deleterious compounds include endotoxins and histamine.[2] Even in the normal state, endotoxin can be found in the rumen contents, and in these situations, it exists without negative systemic effects on the animal.[7] However, endotoxin concentrations will increase in the rumen of animals on a concentrate-based diet.[15] If these animals become acutely acidotic, the acidic environment within the rumen fluid can cause microbial death and release of endotoxin in large quantities all at once.[7] The ability of the normal, intact rumen to absorb endotoxin into the systemic circulation has been questioned, but some researchers have documented endotoxin present in the bloodstream following an acidotic event.[7,16–18]

In addition to endotoxin, histamine is also known to accumulate in the acidotic rumen. Histamine-producing microbes do not exist in large numbers in animals being fed a forage-based ration.[7] However, they proliferate rapidly in cattle on concentrate-based rations, and even more so in an acutely acidic environment. *Allisonella histaminiformans* thrives at low pH, produces large quantities of histamine, and is thought to be the major player in ruminal histamine production.[19] Histamine is not well absorbed by the healthy rumen wall; however, when the ruminal epithelium is damaged as occurs in acidosis, histamine can be absorbed through the rumen wall and into the systemic circulation.[20] Histamine can also be absorbed via the small intestines.[6] There are many effects that histamine is thought to have systemically that may further intensify the symptoms of acute acidosis, including vasodilation and arterioconstriction, and increase vascular permeability.[20,21]

These effects are likely partly responsible for one of the most common sequelae of acidosis in ruminants: laminitis. It is thought that this combination of effects causes blood pressure to increase in capillaries and edema, resulting in swelling, hemorrhage, and even rupture of the vessels.[21] The interruption of blood flow to the tissues in the hoof can thus result in local ischemia and damage to the corium.[21] Laminitis is commonly seen with acidosis in cattle and sheep, but less so in goats.[22] In acidosis of mild severity, animals can experience a transient lameness that seems to resolve following correction of the acidotic event. However, animals experiencing a severe acute case can have more serious lesions, and animals experiencing subacute acidosis can develop subclinical or chronic lesions because of long-term damage to the tissues of the hoof.[21]

CLINICAL SIGNS

The signs of acute rumen acidosis vary according to the type and amount of feed ingested, amount of time since feed ingestion, and severity of physiologic derangements. It is often helpful to classify the manifestations of acidosis into subacute, acute, and peracute forms.[23] In subacute cases, affected animals remain bright, alert, and responsive but may have transient anorexia with signs of mild to moderate dehydration. In these cases, rumen motility is reduced, but diarrhea and signs of abdominal pain are inconsistent.[6,22] In lactating animals, milk production will often be decreased. In some cases, abortions, stillbirths, and premature births may be the only signs seen by caretakers, and the authors have been involved in multiple investigations where abortion storms were the only signs of acidosis noted following the inclusion of bakery waste in the ration of pastured cattle.

In acute cases, affected animals can be found severely obtunded and ataxic. The rumen will usually appear distended, and sloshing of fluid within the rumen is heard on auscultation with abdominal ballottement. Ruminal contractions will be weak to absent.[22] Anorexia will be present, along with profuse, watery, foul-smelling diarrhea. Feces will often be gray in color and may contain bits of undigested grain. In some cases, frank blood may be noted in the feces. In the early stages of disease, rectal temperatures are consistently increased. However, with clinical progression, hypothermia is often detected.[24,25] Tachycardia and tachypnea are present in many cases, with respirations often characterized as shallow.[23] Dehydration and/or hypovolemia are present and are manifested as sinking of the eyes into the orbits, prolonged skin tenting and capillary refill times, delayed jugular filling, weak peripheral pulses, and cold extremities. Neurologic manifestations of disease are seen in many cases and include obtundation, blindness, head pressing, opisthotonus, and altered gait. One particularly useful test is evaluation of the palpebral reflex. There is a very good correlation between the extent of palpebral reflex depression and severity of D-lactic acidosis, and this test might be helpful in categorizing disease severity and monitoring response to therapy.[26,27]

In the peracute form of the disease, animals might be found dead with few or no premonitory signs. In some instances, animals are found recumbent and comatose with the head tucked into the flank. In these severe cases, prognosis is generally poor, and death occurs within a matter of hours.

CLINICAL PATHOLOGY

Multiple diagnostic tests are available to the practitioner evaluating an animal with rumen acidosis. Rumen fluid analysis, complete blood count (CBC), serum or plasma biochemical profiles, blood-gas analysis, and urinalysis have been used to confirm a diagnosis, evaluate disease severity, and assess physiologic derangements. Although not often necessary to confirm a clinical diagnosis, these ancillary diagnostic tests might be of use in determining a prognosis for the individual animal and the degree to which the patient might need to be supported with therapeutic interventions.

Analysis of rumen fluid is one of the most useful diagnostic tests available and should be performed on any animal where rumen acidosis is suspected. Rumen fluid can be collected via passage of an ororumen tube or ruminal paracentesis. As a general rule of thumb, the fluid should be evaluated promptly after collection for color, consistency, odor, pH, and microbial activity (**Table 1**). Normal rumen fluid should be olive or brownish-green and slightly viscous with an aromatic odor. In animals with acidosis, rumen fluid might be milk gray with a putrid odor and watery consistency. In animals on a roughage diet, rumen pH should be 6 to 7, whereas those on high-grain diets might be 5.5 to 6. Regardless, a rumen fluid pH of less than 5.5 is consistent with a diagnosis of rumen acidosis. Microscopically, rumen fluid from animals with acidosis will have decreased numbers and activity of protozoa. Usually, absolute numbers of large and medium protozoa species are decreased. Gram stain can be used to evaluate bacterial diversity and might reveal a shift from gram-negative organisms to a population of predominantly gram-positive organisms.

Hematologic findings in ruminants with acidosis are rarely specific to the condition and generally reflect underlying inflammatory processes. A CBC will often reveal evidence of dehydration and systemic inflammation. Often, animals with acute rumen acidosis will have polycythemia and a neutropenia with a left shift. In animals with longer-standing disturbances, a neutrophilic leukocytosis with hyperfibrinogenemia might be seen.

A serum or plasma biochemical profile might be useful in evaluating organ function, evaluating electrolyte and acid-base homeostasis, and establishing a prognosis. Changes in the biochemical profile are dependent on disease duration and severity

Table 1
Characteristics of rumen fluid in clinical normal ruminants and ruminants with acute rumen acidosis

Parameter	Normal	Rumen Acidosis
Color	Olive to brownish-green	Yellow to gray
Consistency	Viscous	Thin and watery
Odor	Aromatic	Fetid
pH	5.5–7 depending on diet	<5.2
Protozoal activity	Large, medium, and small forms, actively moving	Reduced numbers, little active movement
Gram stain	Predominantly Gram (−)	Predominantly Gram (+)

and include azotemia and hyperphosphatemia, elevations in hepatic enzymes, hyperkalemia, hyperchloremia, mild hypocalcemia, and metabolic acidosis. Azotemia and hyperphosphatemia result from renal compromise associated with hypovolemia and systemic inflammation. Elevations in hepatic enzymes might be reflective of hepatic damage associated with decreased perfusion or bacterial colonization of hepatic tissues. Hyperkalemia is associated with decreased distal tubular flow and accumulation of potassium in circulation.[28] Hyperchloremia and metabolic acidosis are reflective of the accumulation of acid in circulation and titration of the body's buffer systems.

Blood-gas analysis can be helpful in the development of a treatment plan and assessing the severity of acidosis. Ruminants with acidosis will have decreases in plasma pH, elevations in anion gap, and decreases in base excess. In many cases, plasma lactate concentrations are elevated. It is important to note that there might be a discrepancy between plasma lactate concentrations and degree of change in the anion gap and base excess on most commercial blood-gas analyzers. This discrepancy likely reflects the fact that animals with rumen acidosis experience accumulations of both D- and L-lactate in circulation, and most analyzers only detect L-lactate. It is important to remember that D-lactate is an important contributor to the clinical presentation of ruminants with acidosis, and, even though it is not routinely measured, the clinician should not overlook the importance of D-lactate to the pathophysiology of rumen acidosis when designing treatment protocols.

DIAGNOSIS AND PROGNOSIS

Diagnosis of clinical rumen acidosis is based on history of exposure to offending feedstuffs, clinical signs, and ancillary diagnostic tests, particularly rumen fluid analysis. Although the clinical presentation of rumen acidosis can mimic the presentation of other common diseases (mastitis, metritis, peritonitis), the animals' signalment, the lack of signs referable to other body systems, and results of rumen fluid analysis usually can assist the clinician in making an accurate diagnosis and developing an appropriate therapeutic plan. Therefore, a thorough examination of every body system is necessary to rule out other disease syndromes and is an essential component of managing animals with acidosis.

The prognosis for animals with rumen acidosis depends on the duration and severity of clinical signs. Ancillary diagnostic tests play an important role in the assessment of disease severity and development of treatment plans, and their use should be considered if economically feasible. Animals with a blood pH of less than 7.2, rumen pH less than 4.5, severe central nervous system signs, and anuria are less likely to survive than animals with less severe changes. Similarly, animals with peracute disease onset are unlikely to respond to treatment.[23]

TREATMENT

Animals with mild clinical disease might recover with little to no specific care. In animals with more severe clinical disease, specific therapy is necessary and is focused on correction of plasma volume deficits, assessment and treatment of local (rumen) and systemic acid-base disturbances, restoration of a normal rumen microenvironment, and treatment/prevention of potential secondary complications.

Volume deficits are assessed during the initial physical examination, and their severity can be determined in several ways. Although not experimentally validated in mature cattle, the use of eyeball recession has been shown to correlate well with degree of dehydration in calves.[29] The formula for determination of % dehydration based on eyeball recession is as follows:

Degree of recession in millimeters (mm) $\times$ 2 = % dehydration

Thus, an animal with the eyes recessed 5 mm in the orbits would be approximately 10% dehydrated. Other methods of determining fluid deficits include the use of skin tenting times, capillary refill time, jugular filling time, and clinicopathologic variables (**Table 2**). It should be remembered, however, that many of these parameters can be misleading if not interpreted in light of physical examination findings.

Once % dehydration is assessed, the patient's fluid deficits must be estimated and can be done using the following formula:

% dehydration $\times$ body weight (BW) in kg = Fluid deficit in liters (L)

As an example, a 500-kg steer that is 10% dehydrated would require 50 L of fluid to replace existing fluid deficits.

Another consideration when developing a fluid therapy plan for a ruminant with grain overload is assessment of the severity of acid-base disturbances by determining plasma HCO_3^- deficit. The amount of HCO_3^- required to fully replace the total body HCO_3^- deficit can be calculated using the following formula:

0.3 $\times$ BW (kg) $\times$ HCO_3^- deficit = Amount of HCO_3^- required in milliequivalents (mEq)

Again, a 500-kg steer with a plasma HCO_3^- concentration of 5 mEq (HCO_3^- deficit = 25 − 5 = 20) would require 3000 mEq of $NaHCO_3$ to correct the entirety of the calculated deficit.

Dehydration and acidosis are both important considerations for the practitioner when choosing a fluid type for use in a patient with clinical acidosis. Both contribute to morbidity and mortality, and neither factor should be overlooked when choosing a resuscitation fluid. In animals with severe clinical disease, balanced electrolyte solutions should be used to replace existing fluid deficits and provide for maintenance fluid needs. It should be noted that these fluids are usually only being used to address plasma volume deficits and not systemic acid-base disturbances. It is the authors' preference to replace fluid deficits over a period of 24 hours in animals with pure dehydration (sunken eyes and prolonged skin tent with adequate jugular filling and capillary refill time [CRT]). In animals with hypovolemia (prolonged jugular filling, cool extremities, prolonged CRT), the authors use the fluid challenge model whereby 20 mL/kg boluses are given over a 20- to 30-minute period.[30] The patient is reassessed following each bolus and can receive up to 4 boluses before significant fluid overload is a concern. Another option for resuscitation of large ruminants with significant volume deficits is hypertonic saline (HS). HS (7.2%) can be administered at a dose of 4 mL/kg over a period of approximately 10 minutes.[31] It is thought that each milliliter of

Table 2	
Indicators of dehydration and hypovolemia in ruminants with acute rumen acidosis	
Parameter	**Normal Value**
Degree of enophthalmos	<2 mm
Skin tenting time	<1 s
Jugular filling time	Rapid, no delay after compression of vein
Capillary refill time	<2 s
Temperature of extremities (distal limbs, ears) and strength of pulses	Warm to touch, strong pulses

HS will expand plasma volume by 3 to 4 times the amount infused.[32] It is important to remember that the effects of HS are transient and that these solutions must be followed by additional oral or intravenous fluids at a rate of 5 to 10 L per liter of HS infused.[32]

Hypertonic and isotonic solutions of $NaHCO_3$ are commercially available and can be used in conjunction with other fluids to address systemic acidosis. As a general rule of thumb, roughly half the calculated $NaHCO_3$ deficit should be replaced initially, with the remaining half being replaced over the course of 24 to 48 hours. Although the above method may be useful in hospital settings, the diagnostic tests needed to calculate $NaHCO_3$ deficits might not be available in the field. Therefore, protocols have been developed that rely more on a standardized set of recommendations than laboratory diagnostics. One such protocol suggests the use of a 5% solution of $NaHCO_3$, given at a rate of 5 L over 30 minutes for a 450-kg animal, followed by 1.3% $NaHCO_3$ administered at a rate of 150 mL/kg of body weight over 6 to 12 hours.[6] In recent years, many investigators have begun to evaluate 8.4% $NaHCO_3$ solutions for their utility in treating neonatal ruminants with moderate to severe D-lactic acidosis. In these settings, these solutions are safe and effective in treating acidosis and increasing plasma volume.[33,34] Although not specifically evaluated in large ruminants with acute rumen acidosis, 8.4% $NaHCO_3$ might be useful, particularly in field settings where time and resources are limited. $NaHCO_3$ (8.4%) should be administered at a rate of 5 mL/kg of body weight over a period of 10 to 20 minutes.[33,34] Like HS solutions, 8.4% $NaHCO_3$ should be followed with isotonic intravenous or oral fluids to further expand plasma volume and prolong the duration of effect.[33,34]

Restoration of the rumen microenvironment involves removal of acidic rumen contents, administration of rumen buffers, and transfaunation. Removal of abnormal rumen contents can be accomplished in 1 of 2 ways: rumenotomy or rumen lavage. The decision to perform a rumenotomy to remove acidic rumen contents should be made based on the severity of the case, the chances for recovery, and the economic value of the animal. In very severely affected animals of high economic value, rumenotomy can be a highly effective treatment. The surgical techniques to perform the procedure are discussed in detail elsewhere.[25,35] In less severe cases or in animals with lower economic value, removal of the acidic rumen contents can be accomplished by repeated flushing of the rumen with warm water through a large-bore stomach tube. In cattle that are depressed but still standing, this technique allows for a nonsurgical method of removal of rumen contents. This therapy is not well suited to camelids and small ruminants because the diameter of the ororumen tube required precludes passage down the esophagus. With this technique, a large volume of water is pumped into the rumen, and the rumen contents are allowed to flow out by means of pressure and gravity. It is important that an ororumen tube with sufficient diameter be used so that it does not easily become clogged with ingested feedstuffs. Thus, a tube with internal diameter of 1 inch is usually required.[6] Any animals receiving either a rumenotomy or rumen lavage should be transfaunated with rumen fluid taken from a donor on a normal diet. Although the ideal amount of rumen fluid is not known, other investigators have suggested the administration of anywhere from 3 to 10 L in large ruminants.[36] In small ruminants, 2 to 4 L of rumen fluid is usually sufficient.[25]

In animals not undergoing rumenotomy or lavage, oral administration of a buffer is an indispensable and helpful step in correcting ruminal acidosis. A magnesium hydroxide solution is preferable to $NaHCO_3$, because placing $NaHCO_3$ into a highly acidic environment will result in the release of CO_2 and could potentially result in bloat. Magnesium hydroxide should be given at a dose of 1 g/kg of body weight and dissolved in enough water to ensure its dispersal throughout the rumen.[6] It is important to note that the administration of magnesium hydroxide to normal animals is not without consequences.[37] In these patients, magnesium hydroxide will disrupt the rumen microflora, contribute to systemic alkalosis, and cause hypermagnesemia.[37] Thus, rumen acidosis should be confirmed before these agents are administered to any patient.

Numerous sequelae have been associated with clinical rumen acidosis and include polioencephalomalacia (PEM), rumenitis, liver abscessation, laminitis, and vena caval thrombosis. Ancillary therapies are focused on the prevention of longer-term effects of acute ruminal acidosis. One such therapy is the administration of thiamine for the prevention of PEM. The syndrome has been observed in all major domestic ruminant species as well as New World camelids.[9] It is not unusual to see PEM following an acute acidotic event, although the exact mechanism is not fully understood and is discussed in more depth elsewhere.[38] It is thought that PEM following acidosis could be due to the reduction in numbers of thiamine-producing bacteria in the acidic rumen or an increase in the activity of ruminal thiaminases.[38–40] The suggested treatment of PEM in cattle is 10 mg/kg of thiamine given intramuscularly (IM) or subcutaneously, every 8 hours for 3 days in symptomatic animals.[41] The use of dexamethasone, nonsteroidal anti-inflammatory drugs, dimethyl sulfoxide, or diuretics for the treatment and/or prevention of PEM is not supported by the available literature.[40] Another ancillary therapy includes administration of oral or parenteral antimicrobials to prevent liver abscesses and vena caval thrombosis. Unfortunately, the use of antimicrobials in animals with acute acidosis is controversial. Although some have suggested oral administration of penicillin in animals with acidosis, it is not currently recommended because it may have deleterious effects on the rumen microbes and could interfere with reestablishment of a normal bacterial population.[25,35] Nevertheless, parenteral antimicrobials might have some benefit in reducing the development of liver abscesses, and antimicrobials with a spectrum of activity against *F necrophorum* could positively impact patient outcome. The authors routinely recommend the administration of procaine penicillin G at a dose of 22,000 IU/kg IM or ampicillin trihydrate at a dose of 11 mg/kg IM once daily for 3 to 5 days to animals with acute rumen acidosis.

PREVENTION

Prevention of rumen acidosis usually revolves around addressing management practices that precipitate the development of disease in individual animals. In animals unaccustomed to high-concentrate rations, access to easily digestible feedstuffs should be restricted. Sudden changes in feedstuffs should be avoided and, if changes are made, they should be done gradually, as adaptation of the rumen microbes to new feeds might take several weeks. Bunk space must be adequate to allow all animals to access feed without excessive competition. Similarly, animals fed from a bunk should have feed given to them at consistent intervals. If animals are fed from a self-feeder, it is essential to ensure that adequate roughage is available and feed is increased gradually. In addition, monitoring the level of feed in self-feeders is important to ensure animals do not become excessively hungry and gorge themselves when feed is again available. Feed additives such as ionophore antimicrobials, bicarbonate, and limestone might reduce disease severity and incidence when used appropriately.

REFERENCES

1. USDA. Feedlot 2011 "Part IV: Health and health management on US feedlots with a capacity of 1,000 of more head". In: United State Department of

Agriculture, National Animal Health Monitoring System, Washington, DC, editor. 2011. p. 1–100.

2. Nagaraja TG, Lechtenberg KF. Acidosis in feedlot cattle. Vet Clin North Am Food Anim Pract 2007;23:333–50.

3. Smith RA. Impact of disease on feedlot performance: a review. J Anim Sci 1998; 76:272–4.

4. USDA. Cattle on Feed (December 2016). In: United States Department of Agriculture, Washington, DC, National Agricultural Statistics Service, editor. 2016.

5. Owens FN, Secrist DS, Hill WJ, et al. Acidosis in cattle: a review. J Anim Sci 1998; 76:275–86.

6. Radostits OM, Gay CC, Hinchcliff KW, et al. Acute carbohydrate engorgement of ruminants (Ruminal lactic acidosis, rumen overload). In: Radostits OM, Gay CC, Hinchcliff KW, et al, editors. Veterinary medicine. 10th edition. Philadelphia: Saunders Elsevier; 2007. p. 314–25.

7. Nagaraja TG, Titgemeyer EC. Ruminal acidosis in beef cattle: the current microbiological and nutritional outlook. J Dairy Sci 2007;90(Suppl 1):E17–38.

8. Aschenbach JR, Penner GB, Stumpff F, et al. Ruminant Nutrition Symposium: role of fermentation acid absorption in the regulation of ruminal pH. J Anim Sci 2011; 89:1092–107.

9. Smith JA. Noninfectious diseases, metabolic diseases, toxicities, and neoplastic diseases of South American camelids. Vet Clin North Am Food Anim Pract 1989; 5:101–43.

10. Johnson B. Nutritional and dietary interrelationships with diseases of feedlot cattle. Vet Clin North Am Food Anim Pract 1991;7:133–42.

11. Dunlop RH, Hammond PB. D-lactic acidosis of ruminants. Ann N Y Acad Sci 1965;119:1109–32.

12. Garry F, McConnel C. Indigestion in ruminants. In: Smith B, editor. Large animal internal medicine. 4th edition. St Louis (MO): Elsevier; 2009. p. 828–30.

13. Tabaru H, Ikeda K, Kadota E, et al. Effects of osmolality on water, electrolytes and VFAs absorption from the isolated ruminoreticulum in the cow. Jpn J Vet Sci 1990; 52:91–6.

14. Galyean ML, Rivera JD. Nutritionally related disorders affecting feedlot cattle. Can J Anim Sci 2003;83:13–20.

15. Nagaraja TG, Fina LR, Bartley EE, et al. Endotoxic activity of cell-free rumen fluid from cattle fed hay or grain. Can J Microbiol 1978;24:1253–61.

16. Khafipour E, Krause DO, Plaizier JC. A grain-based subacute ruminal acidosis challenge causes translocation of lipopolysaccharide and triggers inflammation. J Dairy Sci 2009;92:1060–70.

17. Gozho GN, Plaizier JC, Krause DO, et al. Subacute ruminal acidosis induces ruminal lipopolysaccharide endotoxin release and triggers an inflammatory response. J Dairy Sci 2005;88:1399–403.

18. Andersen PH, Hesselholt M, Jarlov N. Endotoxin and arachidonic acid metabolites in portal, hepatic and arterial blood of cattle with acute ruminal acidosis. Acta Vet Scand 1994;35:223–34.

19. Garner MR, Flint JF, Russell JB. Allisonella histaminiformans gen. nov., sp. Nov. A novel bacterium that produces histamine, utilizes histidine as its sole energy source, and could play a role in bovine and equine laminitis. Syst Appl Microbiol 2002;25:498–506.

20. Aschenbach JR, Gäbel G. Effect and absorption of histamine in sheep rumen: significance of acidotic epithelial damage. J Anim Sci 2000;78:464–70.

21. Nocek JE. Bovine acidosis: implications on laminitis. J Dairy Sci 1997;80: 1005–28.
22. Van Metre DC, Tyler JW, Stehman SM. Diagnosis of enteric disease in small ruminants. Vet Clin North Am Food Anim Pract 2000;16:87–115.
23. Underwood WJ. Rumen lactic acidosis. Part II. Clinical signs, diagnosis, treatment, and prevention. Comp Cont Ed Pract Vet 1992;14:1265–9.
24. Cebra CK, Cebra ML, Garry FB, et al. Forestomach acidosis in six New World camelids. J Am Vet Med Assoc 1996;208:901–4.
25. Navarre CB, Baird AN, Pugh DG. Diseases of the gastrointestinal system. In: Pugh DG, Baird AN, editors. Sheep and goat medicine. 2nd edition. Maryland Heights (MO): Elsevier Saunders; 2002. p. 71–82.
26. Lorenz I, Gentile A. D-lactic acidosis in neonatal ruminants. Vet Clin North Am Food Anim Pract 2014;30:317–31, v.
27. Lorenz I. Influence of D-lactate on metabolic acidosis and on prognosis in neonatal calves with diarrhoea. J Vet Med A Physiol Pathol Clin Med 2004;51: 425–8.
28. Trefz FM, Constable PD, Sauter-Louis C, et al. Hyperkalemia in neonatal diarrheic calves depends on the degree of dehydration and the cause of the metabolic acidosis but does not require the presence of acidemia. J Dairy Sci 2013;96: 7234–44.
29. Constable PD, Walker PG, Morin DE, et al. Clinical and laboratory assessment of hydration status of neonatal calves with diarrhea. J Am Vet Med Assoc 1998;212: 991–6.
30. Vincent JL, Weil MH. Fluid challenge revisited. Crit Care Med 2006;34:1333–7.
31. Constable PD. Hypertonic saline. Vet Clin North Am Food Anim Pract 1999;15: 559–85.
32. Roussel AJ. Fluid therapy in mature cattle. Vet Clin North Am Food Anim Pract 2014;30:429–39.
33. Koch A, Kaske M. Clinical efficacy of intravenous hypertonic saline solution or hypertonic bicarbonate solution in the treatment of inappetent calves with neonatal diarrhea. J Vet Intern Med 2008;22:202–11.
34. Coskun A, Sen I, Guzelbektes H, et al. Comparison of the effects of intravenous administration of isotonic and hypertonic sodium bicarbonate solutions on venous acid-base status in dehydrated calves with strong ion acidosis. J Am Vet Med Assoc 2010;236:1098–103.
35. Ducharme NG, Fubini SL. Surgery of the ruminant forestomach compartments. In: Fathman EM, editor. Farm animal surgery. St Louis (MO): Saunders Elsevier; 2004. p. 184–96.
36. DePeters EJ, George LW. Rumen transfaunation. Immunol Lett 2014;162:69–76.
37. Smith GW, Correa MT. The effects of oral magnesium hydroxide administration on rumen fluid in cattle. J Vet Intern Med 2004;18:109–12.
38. Gould DH. Polioencephalomalacia. J Anim Sci 1998;76:309–14.
39. Brent BE, Bartley EE. Thiamin and niacin in the rumen. J Anim Sci 1984;59: 813–22.
40. Apley MD. Consideration of evidence for therapeutic interventions in bovine polioencephalomalacia. Vet Clin North Am Food Anim Pract 2015;31:151–61.
41. Cebra CK, Loneragan GH, Gould DH. Polioencephalomalacia (Cerebrocortical necrosis). In: Smith B, editor. Large animal internal medicine. 4th edition. St Louis (MO): Elsevier; 2009. p. 1021–6.

Diagnosis and Management of Subacute Ruminal Acidosis in Dairy Herds

(R) CrossMark

Garrett R. Oetzel, DVM, MS

KEYWORDS

- Dairy cows • Subacute ruminal acidosis • Subclinical acidosis • Chronic acidosis

KEY POINTS

- Subacute ruminal acidosis is diagnosed and prevented at the herd level. Individual cows do not exhibit clinical signs while their ruminal pH is low.
- The pathophysiology of subacute ruminal acidosis is complex, involving both local ruminal effects and systemic inflammation.
- It is difficult to diagnose subacute ruminal acidosis in dairy herds. There is no definitive herd test; instead, information about herd performance, clinical signs, and measured ruminal pH must be integrated.
- Prevention of subacute ruminal acidosis requires excellent feeding management and proper diet formulation.
- Feed additives may reduce (but not eliminate) the risk for subacute ruminal acidosis in dairy herds.

INTRODUCTION

Ruminant animals are adapted to digest and metabolize predominantly forages. Ruminal acidosis may occur when dairy cattle consume diets that provide too much grain. Feeding diets that are progressively higher in grain to dairy cattle tends to increase milk production, even in diets containing up to 75% concentrates.[1] However, short-term gains in milk production may be substantially or completely negated by long-term compromises in cow health when high-grain diets are fed.[2]

Although excessive grain feeding is the main cause of ruminal acidosis in dairy cattle, cows grazing pasture alone are susceptible to ruminal acidosis.[3] Lush grass

Funding Sources: Chr. Hansen Biosystems, Lilly Research Laboratories, and Ridley Block Operations.
The authors have nothing to disclose.
Food Animal Production Medicine Section, Department of Medical Sciences, School of Veterinary Medicine, University of Wisconsin-Madison, 2015 Linden Drive, Madison, WI 53706, USA
E-mail address: gary.oetzel@wisc.edu

from intensively managed pastures can apparently be high enough in rapidly fermentable carbohydrates and low enough in effective fiber to cause ruminal acidosis.[4]

There are 2 major types of ruminal acidosis in dairy cattle: subacute ruminal acidosis (SARA) and acute ruminal acidosis. The definitions for these 2 types of ruminal acidosis come from the beef feedlot industry[5] and have been applied to dairy cattle.[6,7]

SARA is the most common form of ruminal acidosis encountered in dairy herds. It consists of intermittent periods of low ruminal pH that are between acute and chronic in duration. Depressed ruminal pH during SARA self-corrects within a few hours. Affected cows typically exhibit no overt clinical signs when ruminal pH is depressed. However, chronic health problems secondary to rumenitis may appear weeks to months later.

In contrast to SARA, cows with acute ruminal acidosis experience a sudden and uncompensated drop in ruminal pH. They exhibit acute clinical signs and may die.

It is difficult to estimate the prevalence of SARA in dairy herds. The pH of ruminal fluid can be measured; however, spot samples of ruminal pH cannot fully assess the prevalence of SARA because ruminal pH varies considerably with meal patterns.[7] Nonetheless, spot samples are the only practical measure available for estimating the prevalence of SARA in dairy herds. The proportion of cows with ruminal pH ≤ 5.5 using ruminal fluid collected by rumenocentesis has been reported to be 14% in Danish cows, 20% in German cows,[8] and 20% in US cows.[9]

Recognizing the limitations of determining the exact prevalence of SARA, it is apparent that it affects a large number of dairy cattle and causes major economic losses. In addition to the economic losses, SARA also directly impairs cow welfare by increasing the risk for lameness and other chronic health conditions.

PATHOPHYSIOLOGY OF SUBACUTE RUMINAL ACIDOSIS IN DAIRY CATTLE
Low Ruminal pH

Low ruminal pH is the de facto definition of SARA; however, the clinical manifestations of SARA may not be dependent on ruminal pH alone.[10] Harmful metabolites (other than hydrogen ions alone) may be produced by the rumen microbial population depending on the diet fed.[10] Such harmful metabolites may include total ruminal volatile fatty acids (VFA), lactic acid, or ammonia.[11,12] However, alternatives to ruminal pH for defining SARA have not been clearly defined or rigorously evaluated. It is likely safe to assume that low ruminal pH is the major instigator in the pathophysiology of SARA.

Ruminal pH becomes too low because organic acids from ruminal fermentation of carbohydrates accumulate in the rumen. Ruminal pH can be lowered can happen by one (or a combination) of 3 pathways:

- Increased production of organic acids due to overconsumption of ruminally fermentable carbohydrates.
- Insufficient buffering of organic acids in the rumen, which is largely related to effective fiber intake.
- Impaired absorption of organic acids out of the rumen, which is most likely due to rumenitis.

Most of the basic research done on SARA involves the use of cannulated cows with continuous ruminal pH monitoring. By using this system, SARA has been defined as a decline in ruminal pH <5.6 for more than 3 hours per day.[13,14] Other approaches to defining the risk for SARA in research settings include the rate of ruminal pH decrease and the time period when ruminal pH reaches its nadir.[15] Mean daily ruminal pH is not as responsive to dietary changes as the nadir in ruminal pH.[2]

Cattle develop SARA as ruminal pH drops to less than the physiologic threshold of about 5.6. Fortunately, ruminal VFA have a acid dissociation constant of about 4.9 and therefore rapidly shift toward the undissociated (protonated) form as ruminal pH falls below 5.6. This shift removes a free hydrogen ion from the ruminal fluid. It also facilitates VFA absorption across the ruminal epithelium, because VFA are passively absorbed only in the undissociated form.[2]

Unfortunately, gains in VFA absorption at ruminal pH <5.6 can be offset by lactate production. At high growth rates (triggered by high levels of starch and sugars in the rumen), *Streptococcus bovis* begins to ferment glucose to lactate instead of VFA. Lactate has a much lower dissociation constant than VFA (3.9 vs 4.8) and therefore depresses ruminal pH much more rapidly. Very low ruminal pH creates a niche for lactobacilli that produce even more lactate.[16] Ruminal lactate also is poorly absorbed from the rumen because it is much less dissociated than VFA. Retention of lactate in the rumen further contributes to a rapid downward spiral in ruminal pH.[2]

Additional adaptive responses are invoked as ruminal pH declines and lactate production begins. Lactate-utilizing bacteria, such as *Megasphaera elsdenii* and *Selenomonas ruminantium*, proliferate and convert lactate to other VFA, which are then easily protonated and absorbed. Most of the lactate produced can be metabolized by these bacteria.[17]

Increased Ruminal Lactate

The depression of ruminal pH during SARA is apparently due to the accumulation of VFA and is not caused primarily by lactate accumulation.[2] Nonetheless, frequent measurement of ruminal lactate during the day under conditions associated with SARA will reveal transient spikes of ruminal lactate between about 10 and 40 mM.[1,18] The exact role of these transient lactate spikes is not known, but they probably contribute to lowered ruminal pH.

Increased Ruminal Valerate

Valerate is produced in the rumen by lactolytic bacteria in the presence of lactate.[17] High concentrations of ruminal valerate may indicate a prior occurrence of SARA.[19]

Reduced Dry Matter Intake

SARA is self-limiting largely because it depresses dry matter intake. Depressed intake reduces acid production in the rumen and allows rapid restoration of normal ruminal pH. Potential causes of intake depression include decreased frequency and amplitude of ruminal contractions, increased ruminal lactic acid concentrations, increased ruminal osmotic pressure, and inflammation of the ruminal epithelium.[20]

Feed Ingredient Selection

Reduced dry matter intake is not the cow's only option for self-correction of low ruminal pH. Cows are able to alter their diet preference for higher physically effective fiber and slower starch fermentability during a bout of SARA.[21]

Cow Behavior

Bouts of ruminal acidosis have little overall effect on measures of cow behavior, such as standing time, lying time, or feeding time. Rumination activity decreases slightly during bouts of ruminal acidosis.[22]

Inflammation

Gram-negative bacteria in the rumen are particularly sensitive to low pH. During periods of SARA, they may die and release endotoxins; the amount of endotoxin released depends on type of diet fed and the gram-negative bacterial populations present.[14] Bacterial endotoxin release triggers a local inflammatory response in the rumen. The lipopolysaccharide (LPS) from these endotoxins can then translocate into systemic circulation and trigger a systemic inflammatory response.[14] The metabolic consequences of systemic LPS are far reaching and include inhibited casein synthesis in the mammary gland,[23] inflammation in the uterus leading to endometritis,[24] and hepatocellular damage.[25]

Markers of inflammation such as blood concentrations of acute phase proteins (haptoglobin and serum amyloid A) may be increased during periods of ruminal acidosis.[26,27] Different methods of SARA induction result in different acute phase protein responses.[14]

It should be noted that not all cows with experimentally induced SARA have detectable LPS in the bloodstream[28] and that bacterial endotoxin from the rumen may not be the sole cause of the inflammatory response associated with SARA.[14] Blood haptoglobin may be elevated by other infectious conditions such as mastitis[29] or metritis.[30] Increases in haptoglobin following SARA could be the result of secondary infections, such as liver abscesses or pneumonia, instead of being a direct result of SARA.

Histamine is another inflammatory mediator that may be produced during SARA. Histamine has been traditionally associated with the pathogenicity of SARA[31]; however, precise information about the role of histamine in the pathogenesis of SARA is lacking. Histamine may be produced in the rumen during periods of low ruminal pH.[32] Permeability of the ruminal epithelium to histamine is low, except during periods of low ruminal pH, which apparently compromise epithelial integrity and allow for histamine absorption.[33]

Reduced Feed Efficiency

SARA decreases feed efficiency because cellulolytic bacteria in the rumen are very sensitive to low ruminal pH.[34] The extent of the reduction in fiber digestibility during SARA is substantial, between about 20% and 25%.[35] Reduced fiber digestibility directly reduces herd profitability and increases the environmental footprint of milk production.

Milk Fat Depression

SARA may cause milk fat depression; however, this effect is inconsistent and complex.[14,18] Low ruminal pH apparently causes milk fat depression by inhibiting bacteria responsible for fatty acid biohydrogenation in the rumen.[14] Incomplete biohydrogenation of these fatty acids increases the amount of absorbed trans-fatty acids.[36] Longer-term SARA may be necessary before milk fat depression is evident.[14]

Other important causes of milk fat depression include overfeeding of unsaturated fats and monensin supplementation. All of these causes of milk fat depression are interrelated because they all affect the same pathway: incomplete ruminal biohydrogenation of fatty acids.[36]

Individual Cow Susceptibility to Subacute Ruminal Acidosis

Individual animals have remarkably different susceptibilities to ruminal acidosis.[11] It has been shown that cows known to be more susceptible to SARA sort against long particles in the diet.[37] There are probably other differences between cows with high and low susceptibilities to SARA.

Rumenitis

Ruminal epithelial cells are not protected by mucus (as abomasal cells are), so they may be vulnerable to the chemical damage by excessive acidity.[2] Low ruminal pH has been associated with inflammation of the ruminal epithelium (rumenitis), which may advance to erosion and ulceration.[6] Maintaining the integrity of the ruminal epithelium is crucial because it serves as the only protective layer between the rumen environment and portal circulation.[38] Unfortunately, dramatic structural changes to the ruminal epithelium occur within a few days of an acidotic insult.[39]

Ruminal acidosis weakens cellular adhesion between cells in the ruminal epithelium, which allows transmural migration of rumen microbes into portal circulation. This leakage leads to a variety of secondary infections, which are described in later discussion. Weakened adhesion between cells may also increase translocation of endotoxins into the bloodstream.[14]

Parakeratosis (thickening of the stratum corneum of the ruminal epithelium) may be the result of chronic rumenitis.[40] Parakeratosis is clinically important because it decreases VFA absorption[41] and may predispose affected animals to future SARA episodes.

Hindgut Acidosis

Hindgut acidosis occurs when excessive carbohydrate fermentation in the large intestine leads to an accumulation of organic acids.[42] Conditions of excessive intake of fermentable carbohydrates may cause both ruminal acidosis and hindgut acidosis. The presence of hindgut acidosis implies that not all of the fermentable carbohydrates consumed by the cow were actually fermented in the rumen; some passed through to the hindgut and were fermented to organic acids there. Several studies have reported reduced fecal pH during induced SARA.[43,44]

As for ruminal acidosis, hindgut acidosis may cause a breach in the gut epithelium that allows for systemic entry of bacteria, toxins, or histamine. Absorption of these metabolites further contributes to systemic inflammation and perhaps laminitis.[42]

Diarrhea

Diarrhea, frothy feces, and the presence of mucin casts in the feces have been clinically associated with SARA.[45] Mucin or fibrin casts found in feces may be a secondary response to hindgut sloughing of epithelial cells followed by secretion of mucous and fibrin to protect the injured tissue.[46]

Changes in fecal consistency are not typically noted in SARA induction studies, even when fecal pH is very low.[18] The reasons for this are unclear. This finding suggests that something else may be responsible for diarrhea that is often attributed to SARA. One possibility is that hindgut protein is the more likely culprit when herd-wide diarrhea is observed without an apparent infectious cause. Soluble proteins in the hindgut (whether of microbial or dietary origin) cannot be absorbed from the hindgut. As a result, they may remain osmotically active there and cause diarrhea. In contrast, organic acids produced by microbial fermentation of carbohydrates in the hindgut can be absorbed.

Altered Ruminal Microflora

SARA upsets the complex balance of microbes in the rumen. The ruminal bacterial community composition changes rapidly during SARA challenge models; different changes likely occur when cattle are exposed to repeated bouts of SARA over a longer time period.[47] Of particular importance during SARA is a loss of diversity in both ruminal and epimural bacterial communities.[47,48] It is particularly important that major fiber-digesting species are particularly sensitive to low ruminal pH.[49] Cows exposed to repeated bouts of SARA have different microbial responses and may be less capable of responding to future challenges to rumen stability.[47]

Escherichia coli bacteria are particularly capable of triggering an inflammatory response in cattle.[14] High starch feeding increases the number of *E coli* throughout the digestive tract.[50] Of particular concern is enterohemorrhagic *E coli* 0157:H7, which is an important human pathogen and is shed in higher numbers with high-grain feeding.[51]

Liver Abscess Formation

Liver abscesses are a common complication of SARA. They are caused by bacterial leakage across damaged ruminal epithelium. Portal blood flow then carries the bacteria to the liver, where they may establish a new infection that is walled off into an abscess.

A slaughter survey of predominantly Holsteins reported 32% liver abscesses, 57% of which were categorized as severe abscesses. In the same survey, severe ruminal lesions and rumenitis scars were observed in 10% of the cows, and 3% of the cows had short or denuded ruminal papillae.[52] These findings illustrate a key feature of SARA, namely that the ruminal epithelium can heal fairly quickly after an acidotic insult, but secondary problems such as liver abscesses that are due to bacterial leakage may persist considerably longer.

Other Infectious Diseases Secondary to Rumenitis

If the ruminal bacteria clear the liver (or if bacteria from liver infections are released into circulation), they may colonize the lungs, heart valves, kidneys, or joints. The resulting pneumonia, endocarditis, pyelonephritis, and arthritis are all chronic inflammatory diseases that are difficult to diagnose ante mortem. Caudal vena cava syndrome can cause hemoptysis and peracute deaths due to massive pulmonary hemorrhage in cows that are affected with SARA. In these cases, septic emboli from liver abscesses lead to lung infections that ultimately invade pulmonary vessels and cause their rupture.[6]

Lameness

SARA appears to interact with time standing on concrete to cause lameness problems in herds.[45] Lameness may be associated with SARA in grazing herds as well.[53]

The mechanisms by which SARA increases the risk for lameness are not well understood. A direct effect of systemic LPS on capillaries in the hoof has been proposed[54]; however, this seems to be unlikely because SARA may increase free LPS in the rumen but not in peripheral circulation.[27]

Laminitis in horses can be caused by activation of metalloproteinase enzymes within the lamellar structure of the hoof. Exotoxins produced by *S bovis* during periods of hindgut acidosis are responsible for activating the metalloproteinases.[55] Whether this pathway occurs in cattle has not been proven. However, laminitis in cattle has been experimentally induced by oral dosing with oligofructose,[56] which is a carbohydrate that may be extensively fermented in the hindgut.[57] It is not clear whether oligofructose sufficiently escapes ruminal fermentation to be presented to the hindgut of cattle.

Reduced Body Condition Score

Considering the association of SARA with lameness and chronic inflammatory conditions, it seems intuitive that cows suffering from bouts of SARA would have reduced body condition score. A survey of Dutch herds reported that cows with low ruminal pH lost more body condition over the calving period.[58] A German survey similarly reported that cows with low ruminal pH had lower body condition scores compared with cows having normal ruminal pH.[8] This association may not always be present; there was no association of body condition score with SARA classification for grazing herds in an Australian study.[53]

Impaired Immune Function

Given that SARA has the potential to stimulate a chronic inflammatory response and decrease feed intake, it is logical that it would contribute to immune suppression and increased susceptibility to other infectious diseases. Clear evidence for this is sparse, however. One study reported that SARA induction increased the risk for mastitis and reduced milk quality.[59]

CLINICAL SIGNS IN DAIRY HERDS AFFECTED WITH SUBACUTE RUMINAL ACIDOSIS

Dairy herds affected with SARA may have a high prevalence of thin cows (despite relatively high energy density in the diets), a high prevalence of lame cows (especially if the main types of lameness are secondary to laminitis), and lower than expected milk fat percentage. It is not typical to find all of these signs present in a single herd, unless SARA has been long-standing and severe.

DIAGNOSIS OF SUBACUTE RUMINAL ACIDOSIS IN DAIRY HERDS
Evaluating Clinical Signs Associated with Subacute Ruminal Acidosis

Two of the key features of SARA (transient depression in dry matter intake and reduced milk yield) cannot be practically determined in affected herds. The condition is usually long-standing at the herd level, and individual cows may be cycling at different times through periods of low ruminal pH followed by recovery.

Ruminal pH

Although ruminal pH is the best test currently for diagnosing SARA, it has major limitations and is most useful for finding severely affected herds. Ruminal pH may vary from day to day and time of day within a herd. Thus, single samplings of a group of cows are vulnerable to error. Methods that allow for continuous monitoring of ruminal pH for several days are preferred but are not practical for routine use in diagnosing SARA in dairy herds.

Measuring Ruminal pH via Fluid Collected by Ororuminal Probe

The pH of ruminal fluid collected via an ororuminal probe may be contaminated by saliva and thus have a considerably higher pH than ruminal fluid collected through a ruminal cannula.[60] Several recent studies have reported a more favorable comparison between orally collected samples and samples taken via ruminal cannula.[61,62] For best results, insert the ororuminal tube to a depth of about 200 cm so that the end of the sampling tube reaches the central rumen.[63]

Measuring Ruminal pH via Fluid Collected by Rumenocentesis

A technique for determining ruminal fluid pH via a sample collected by rumenocentesis has been described in detail.[64] Rumenocentesis was more sensitive than orally collected ruminal fluid for diagnosing low ruminal pH.[60] As for oral ruminal fluid collection, this technique provides only a spot sample for ruminal pH.

In brief, the technique for collecting ruminal fluid by rumenocentesis involves restraining the cow well, inserting a 1.2-mm-diameter (16-gauge) needle approximately 100 mm long (4 inch) into the rumen, and aspirating 1 mL of ruminal fluid. A field pH meter can then be used to determine the pH of the fluid. The procedure causes only mild stress to the cows and does not affect dry matter intake or milk yield.[65] The technique is done without local anesthetic, which results in no more stress to the cow than injecting a local anesthetic before inserting the needle into the rumen.[65]

The site of ruminal fluid collection may influence the risk for complications following the procedure. Puncture into the dorsal sac of the rumen caused no apparent complications.[65] However, fluid collected from the dorsal sac may have a higher pH because of variable amounts of saliva contamination.[63] The initial description of the rumenocentesis procedure involves puncture into the ventral sac (at the level of the stifle).[64] The investigators reported only occasional subcutaneous abscesses from this procedure.

Severe complications were reported when rumenocentesis was performed with a very large needle (1.8 mm or 13 gauge), and a relatively large volume (10 mL) of ruminal fluid was collected from the ventral sac of the rumen.[66] This approach to rumenocentesis is not recommended.

A pH meter should be used for determining the pH of ruminal fluid. Each time the meter is used, it must be first calibrated with pH 4 and pH 7 buffers. Test paper strips for pH are not suitable for measuring ruminal pH, because the color of the ruminal fluid may interfere with the interpretation of the color change on the strip.

The pH of ruminal fluid samples may be evaluated immediately after collection. Alternatively, the ruminal fluid may be stored in a capped syringe (with all of the air excluded) before pH analysis.

The minimal sample size for ruminal pH evaluation is 12 animals per diet.[9] If 3 or more of the 12 cows tested have a ruminal pH ≤ 5.5, then the group is considered to be at high risk for SARA, and the diet should be modified to reduce the risk for SARA. This testing scheme works best for herds with high (>30%) or low (<15%) prevalence of cows with low ruminal pH. Herds with intermediate prevalence (16.7%–33.3%) of low ruminal pH may require a greater sample size to be more likely to be classified correctly, or may require that other diagnostic indicators of SARA be more carefully considered. Immediate dietary intervention is not critical in herds with intermediate prevalence, so it is not unreasonable to take some additional time to gather more information.

Time relative to feeding has a major effect on ruminal pH. The purpose of herd-based ruminal pH testing is to identify cows with low ruminal pH, whenever it might occur. Therefore, sampling should be done around the time of the expected lowest point (nadir). In component-fed herds, the nadir in ruminal pH occurs about 2 to 4 hours after feeding. In total mixed ration (TMR)-fed herds, the nadir in ruminal pH occurs about 6 to 12 hours after feeding.[18]

Measuring Ruminal pH via Indwelling pH Sensors

Indwelling wireless pH sensors are used in research studies with SARA. The advantages of wireless sensors are that they can be administered to noncannulated cows, allowing them to eat and behave as they normally would throughout the day while their ruminal pH is recorded. Such sensors have the potential for use in commercial herds if the cost of the sensors can be lowered and their longevity improved.

Wireless sensors for ruminal pH monitoring must also account for the location in which pH is measured. Most ruminal pH sensors reside in the reticulum. However, recommended pH thresholds for SARA are derived from measurements taken from liquid usually collected from the ventral sac of the rumen. Reticular pH is typically about 0.2 pH units higher than pH from fluid collected from the ventral sac of the rumen.[67] However, a more detailed evaluation reported that the difference between ruminal and reticular pH varies across week of lactation. Because of this variation, the investigators could not offer a fixed conversion factor to make pH measurements in the reticulum comparable with those in the rumen.[68]

Milk Fatty Acid Profile

Low ruminal pH alters the ruminal environment such that biohydrogenation is altered to favor the formation of specific fatty acids.[69,70] However, there are no commercially available tests for these specific milk fatty acids.

Rumination Measurements

Cows consuming diets that are very low in effective fiber may have a low percentage of cows ruminating at a given time.[2] Approximately 40% of cows not eating should be ruminating at any time of the day.[71] Cows were observed to have reduced rumination time during a bout of induced SARA; however, the differences were not large enough to be detectable in single herd observation.[22] The use of automated sensors for detecting rumination activity may provide some indication of herd-level SARA; however, this hypothesis has not been evaluated.

Acute Phase Proteins

Acute phase protein tests help validate the role that inflammation may play in SARA; however, they are not unique responses to SARA and are not practical tools for diagnosing SARA on dairy farms.

Fecal pH

Fecal pH often mirrors ruminal pH following a lag time of about 12 to 18 hours.[44] Visible changes in fecal appearance are not necessarily a feature of very low fecal pH. Because ruminal pH reaches its nadir about 8 to 14 hours after the morning feeding, fecal pH would typically need to be measured in the middle of the night in order to be reflective of ruminal pH. This timing of measurement is not inherently practical, but could have utility in diagnosing SARA in herds. There has been no formal evaluation of this approach to diagnosing SARA in herds.

Ultrasound

Repeated bouts of SARA cause thickening of the ruminal mucosa.[19] Transabdominal ultrasonography may have value in identifying this thickening and allowing for a noninvasive diagnosis of SARA. One study suggested that the best site for evaluating thickness of the ruminal mucosa was at an intersection of a horizontal line going through the costochondral junction and a vertical line coming from the third lumbar vertebra.[72] This approach has not been validated for herd-level diagnosis of SARA but could have potential.

PREVENTION OF SUBACUTE RUMINAL ACIDOSIS IN DAIRY HERDS

There is no diagnosis or treatment of SARA in individual dairy cows. The diagnosis is made at the herd level, and prevention strategies are applied at the herd level.

Feeding a Total Mixed Ration

Cows fed a TMR are at lower risk for ruminal acidosis compared with cows fed their diet as separate components.[2] Using a TMR to deliver the diet to cattle reduces the size of grain meals and forces the inclusion of forage with every meal. The main difficulty with component feeding is that it creates large grain meals that may dramatically drop ruminal pH after feeding.

Excellent Feeding Management

The starting point for prevention of SARA is limiting the size of individual meals and increasing the frequency of meals. When given the chance, dairy cows have some ability to self-regulate their ruminal pH. However, they cannot regulate their own ruminal pH unless they have adequate access to eating space so that cows can eat when they want and consume the amount they want at each meal. It also requires extremely consistent delivery of feed at the same time (and at the same time relative to milking, because cattle often eat their biggest meals following milking).

Feed must also be available at the bunk whenever cows wish to eat meals. Dairy cattle groups are commonly fed for ad libitum intake (typically a 5% daily feed refusal) in order to maximize potential dry matter intake and milk yield. However, slightly limiting intake in dairy cattle at high risk for SARA would in theory reduce their risk of periodic overconsumption and SARA. Feed efficiency might also be improved. This approach has been successfully used in beef feedlots. However, dairy cow groups are much more dynamic than feedlot groups, making it considerably more challenging for dairy cattle feeders to slightly limit intakes without letting the feed bunks be empty too long. Even modest bouts of excessive feed restriction can cause cows to subsequently consume meals that are too large.

Providing Adequate Effective Fiber in the Diet

An important goal of effective dairy cow nutrition is to feed as much concentrate as possible, in order to maximize production, without causing ruminal acidosis. This task is difficult and challenging because the indications of feeding excessive amounts of fermentable carbohydrates (decreased dry matter intake and milk production) are very similar to the results from feeding excessive fiber (again, decreased dry matter intake and milk production). An important distinction is that even slightly overfeeding fermentable carbohydrates causes chronic health problems, whereas slightly underfeeding fermentable carbohydrates does not compromise cow health.

Much attention has been devoted to determining optimal proportions of different carbohydrates (both fiber and nonfiber carbohydrates) in dairy cattle. The specifics of dietary formulation for fiber adequacy are usually handled by dairy nutritionists and not by veterinarians per se. In brief, key aspects of fiber adequacy for lactating cow diets are as follows:

- Neutral detergent fiber (NDF) in the diet organic matter: 30% to 32% of diet dry matter
- Physically effective NDF (peNDF): 21% to 24% of diet dry matter, where peNDF is defined as NDF that is retained on top of a 4-mm sieve using 2-dimensional wet sieving[73]
- Long forage particles (defined as particles retained on the top of a 19-mm screen using the Penn State Forage Particle Separator): 7% to 12% of the total particles
- Starch: 22 to 26 of diet dry matter
- Sugars (as determined by water extraction): 4% to 8% of diet dry matter

Meeting these criteria on their own is not yet sufficient for defining fiber adequacy. The physical form of grains can be just as important as their chemical composition in determining how rapidly and completely they are fermented in the rumen. Grains that are finely ground, steam-flaked, extruded, or very wet will ferment more rapidly and completely in the rumen than unprocessed or dry grains, even if their chemical composition is identical. Similarly, starch from wheat or barley is more rapidly and completely fermented in the rumen than starch from corn. Particle size analysis of grains is a useful adjunct test when assessing the risk for SARA in a dairy herd. Very finely ground grains, especially if they are moist, will have an increased rate of fermentation in the rumen and increase the risk for SARA. Guidelines for evaluating grain processing have been reviewed in detail elsewhere.[74]

There are many subtle interactions between the different measures of fiber adequacy in dairy cattle diets. For example, fiber should be increased when highly fermentable grains are fed.[2] When particle length of the diet is short, chemical fiber (NDF) can be increased to compensate.[75]

Diets with excessive (over about 15%) long forage particles may contain too many long particles that are unpalatable and sortable, thus paradoxically increasing the risk for SARA.[2] Sorting of the long particles occurs soon after feed delivery, causing the cows to consume a diet that is low in physically effective fiber after feeding. The diet consumed later in the feeding period is then excessively high in physically effective fiber and low in energy. Socially dominant cows are particularly susceptible to SARA in this scenario, because they are likely to consume more of the fine TMR particles soon after feed delivery. Cows lower on the pecking order then consume a very low energy diet.

Sorting of long particles during the feed-out period can be evaluated by conducting sequential analysis of the TMR bunk samples at differing times after feeding. A detailed protocol for accomplished this has been published.[74] Potential remedies for excessive TMR sorting include processing dry hay correctly before adding it to the TMR, adding less hay to the TMR, switching to higher quality hay, adding water to the TMR until it is about 45% dry matter, including liquid molasses in the TMR, feeding small amounts of TMR more frequently, increasing daily feed refusals, and providing sufficient eating space so that all of the cows can eat at the same time.

Once cows develop SARA, they may sort toward longer particles in an effort to attenuate their ruminal acidosis.[76] Unfortunately, there is no practical means of making it more feasible for cows to select longer forage particles during periods of SARA. Offering free-choice hay outside of the TMR is not recommended, because it could set cows up to develop more SARA by expressing a preference not to consume the hay when ruminal pH is normal.

Maximizing Ruminal Buffering

Ruminant animals have a highly developed system for buffering the organic acids produced by ruminal fermentation of carbohydrates. Although the total effect of buffering on ruminal pH is relatively small, it can still account for the margin between health and disease in dairy cows fed large amounts of fermentable carbohydrates.

Endogenous buffers are produced by the cow and secreted into the rumen with saliva flow during eating and ruminating. Endogenous buffering is maximized when cows are provided adequate long particles in the diet, as described above.

Dietary buffering represents the inherent buffering capacity of the diet and is largely explained by dietary cation-anion difference (DCAD).[2] Diets high in Na and K relative to Cl and S have a higher DCAD and promote higher ruminal pH.[77] Buffers such as $NaHCO_3$ and K_2CO_3 are added to diets to increase DCAD beyond the inherent

DCAD of the diet ingredients. Optimal DCAD (expressed as $[(Na + K) - (Cl + S)]$) in lactating diets is about 275 to 450 mEq/kg of diet dry matter. Adding more dietary buffers to the point that DCAD exceeds 450 mEq/kg results in no further improvement in dry matter intake or milk yield.[77]

Provision of Free-Choice Buffers

It is widely assumed that dairy cattle will consume additional free-choice buffers during periods of SARA. However, numerous well-designed experiments indicate that this is not the case.[78,79] The provision of free-choice buffers or buffer blocks should not be discouraged, because there could be individual cows that might benefit from their availability. It is important, however, not to rely on free-choice buffers to be an integral part of dietary buffering. They should be considered supplemental only.

Although many nutritionists monitor free-choice buffer intake as a means of determining whether a herd is going through a period of SARA, this practice is not supported by experimental evidence. Free-choice buffer intake may vary considerably over time within a herd, but it appears that unknown factors other than ruminal pH are responsible.

Allowing for Adequate Ruminal Adaptation to Higher Concentrate Diets

In theory, cows in early lactation should be particularly susceptible to SARA if they are poorly prepared for the lactation diet they will receive. Ruminal adaptation to diets high in fermentable carbohydrates apparently has 2 key aspects: microbial adaptation (particularly the lactate-utilizing bacteria, which grow more slowly than the lactate-producing bacteria) and ruminal papillae length (longer papillae promote greater VFA absorption and thus lower ruminal pH).[40]

Dairy cows have an increase in ruminal papillae mass at 10 days after calving compared with the precalving period.[80] There was no further increase in mass from 10 to 22 days after calving. An increase in ruminal papillae mass may explain why ruminal pH can increase during the first 3 weeks after calving despite increased dry matter intake.[81]

The practical impacts of ruminal adaptation may be small or even inconsequential in dairy herds, particularly when cows are fed a TMR after calving.[82] Of more practical significance is the need to prevent periods of feed deprivation. These periods of feed deprivation lead to very high ruminal pH (approximately 7.0–7.5), which inhibits the growth of lactate using bacteria and leaves the ruminal microbial populations more susceptible to acidosis.[2]

Besides disrupting ruminal microbial balance, feed deprivation causes cattle to consume large meals when feed is reintroduced, creating a double effect that can lower ruminal pH very rapidly.[2]

Overview of Feed Additives for the Prevention of Subacute Ruminal Acidosis

The keys to lowering the risk for SARA are lowering the intake of fermentable carbohydrate and enhancing ruminal buffering. Additional nutritional interventions that might prevent SARA without limiting grain feeding are highly desirable. No feed additives are able to completely attenuate the risk for SARA.[83] Their use should also be considered supplemental to the feeding management and dietary formulation strategies presented above. Judicious use of feed additives to reduce the risk for SARA is warranted because it is very costly and very difficult to monitor.

Increasing Dietary Sugars

Feeding sugars as a partial replacement for dietary starch lowers the risk for SARA. Because sugars ferment more rapidly to VFA in the rumen than starches, it is not intuitive that feeding relatively more sugars would increase ruminal pH. The mechanism or mechanisms for this desirable response are unclear but appear to be at least partially mediated by increased organic acid absorption.[84] Many dairy diets require the addition of supplemental sugars in order to meet the minimum requirement of about 4% diet dry matter as sugars.

Yeast Supplementation

Yeast supplementation may reduce the risk for SARA, particularly during abrupt changes from high-forage to high-grain diets.[85] Mechanisms proposed for this benefit are mainly focused on optimizing fiber digestion.[85,86]

Monensin

Monensin, an ionophore antibiotic, may improve ruminal pH because it inhibits most lactate-producing ruminal bacteria while leaving lactate consuming bacteria unaffected. However, monensin has not been shown to increase ruminal pH during periods of SARA in dairy cattle.[81,87] Perhaps monensin is effective in reducing the risk for SARA only when lactate production is substantial.[88]

Dicarboxylic Acids

The dicarboxylic acids aspartate, fumarate, and malate may help reduce the risk for SARA by increasing ruminal lactic acid uptake and favoring production of propionate.[89] The mechanism of action is via enhanced lactate utilization by *Sruminantium*. Malate has the most potent effects. Inclusion of malate as a feed additive is cost-prohibitive; however, certain alfalfa varieties may be very rich in malate.[89] A fumarate malate–blended feed supplement has been developed and shown to attenuate the drop in ruminal pH during an SARA induction model.[90]

Flavonoids and Essential Oils

Flavonoids and essential oils are plant-derived compounds that may modify rumen fermentation. Flavonoids appear to improve fermentation and increase the numbers of lactate-consuming microbes in the rumen.[91] Essential oils may modify rumen fermentation, depending on the specific oil used.[92] A blend of essential oils and polyphenol attenuated the drop in ruminal pH and the inflammatory response during an SARA induction model.[90]

SUMMARY

SARA is a challenging disorder to recognize and prevent in dairy herds. There is no consensus as to the exact cause of SARA, although depressed ruminal pH is probably the main factor. The pathophysiology of SARA is complex and variable, and the clinical manifestations do not occur until weeks or months later. There is no single, definitive test for SARA, yet a careful integration of clinical and diagnostic data should lead to correct decisions. Monitoring SARA is difficult and imprecise because it is impractical to continuously monitor ruminal pH. Prevention of SARA requires careful attention to feeding management and diet formulation. There is no singularly effective feed additive to prevent SARA, but judicious use of available products can be helpful. Despite these many challenges, efforts to understand and manage this disease are worthwhile. The health, welfare, productivity, and environmental impact of dairy cows greatly depend on how well SARA is managed in dairy herds.

REFERENCES

1. Kennelly JJ, Robinson B, Khorasani GR. Influence of carbohydrate source and buffer on rumen fermentation characteristics, milk yield, and milk composition in early-lactation Holstein cows. J Dairy Sci 1999;82(11):2486–96.
2. Krause KM, Oetzel GR. Understanding and preventing subacute ruminal acidosis in dairy herds: a review. Anim Feed Sci Tech 2006;126:215–36.
3. O'Grady L, Doherty ML, Mulligan FJ. Subacute ruminal acidosis (SARA) in grazing Irish dairy cows. Vet J 2008;176(1):44–9.
4. Westwood CT, Bramley E, Lean IJ. Review of the relationship between nutrition and lameness in pasture-fed dairy cattle. N Z Vet J 2003;51(5):208–18.
5. Owens FN, Secrist DS, Hill WJ, et al. Acidosis in cattle: a review. J Anim Sci 1998; 76(1):275–86.
6. Nordlund KV, Garrett EF, Oetzel GR. Herd-based rumenocentesis: a clinical approach to the diagnosis of subacute rumen acidosis. Compend Contin Educ Pract Vet 1995;17(8):S48–56.
7. Garrett EF, Pereira MN, Nordlund KV, et al. Diagnostic methods for the detection of subacute ruminal acidosis in dairy cows. J Dairy Sci 1999;82(6):1170–8.
8. Kleen JL, Upgang L, Rehage J. Prevalence and consequences of subacute ruminal acidosis in German dairy herds. Acta Vet Scand 2013;55:48.
9. Oetzel GR. Monitoring and testing dairy herds for metabolic disease. Vet Clin North Am Food Anim Pract 2004;20(3):651–74.
10. Calsamiglia SB, Blanch M, Ferret A, et al. Is subacute ruminal acidosis a pH related problem? Causes and tools for its control. Anim Feed Sci Tech 2012; 172:42–50.
11. Golder HM, Celi P, Lean IJ. Ruminal acidosis in a 21-month-old Holstein heifer. Can Vet J 2014;55(6):559–64.
12. Bramley E, Lean IJ, Fulkerson WJ, et al. The definition of acidosis in dairy herds predominantly fed on pasture and concentrates. J Dairy Sci 2008;91(1):308–21.
13. AlZahal O, Kebreab E, France J, et al. A mathematical approach to predicting biological values from ruminal pH measurements. J Dairy Sci 2007;90(8): 3777–85.
14. Plaizier JC, Krause DO, Gozho GN, et al. Subacute ruminal acidosis in dairy cows: the physiological causes, incidence and consequences. Vet J 2008; 176(1):21–31.
15. Dragomir C, Sauvant D, Peyraud JL, et al. Meta-analysis of 0 to 8 h post-prandial evolution of ruminal pH. Animal 2008;2(10):1437–48.
16. Russell JB, Hino T. Regulation of lactate production in Streptococcus bovis: a spiraling effect that contributes to rumen acidosis. J Dairy Sci 1985;68(7): 1712–21.
17. Counotte GHM, Prins RA. Regulation of lactate metabolism in the rumen. Vet Res Commun 1981;5(2):101–15.
18. Krause KM, Oetzel GR. Inducing subacute ruminal acidosis in lactating dairy cows. J Dairy Sci 2005;88(10):3633–9.
19. Enemark JM. The monitoring, prevention and treatment of sub-acute ruminal acidosis (SARA): a review. Vet J 2008;176(1):32–43.

20. Desnoyers M, Giger-Reverdin S, Duvaux-Ponter C, et al. Modeling of off-feed periods caused by subacute acidosis in intensive lactating ruminants: application to goats. J Dairy Sci 2009;92(8):3894–906.

21. Maulfair DD, McIntyre KK, Heinrichs AJ. Subacute ruminal acidosis and total mixed ration preference in lactating dairy cows. J Dairy Sci 2013;96(10):6610–20.

22. DeVries TJ, Beauchemin KA, Dohme F, et al. Repeated ruminal acidosis challenges in lactating dairy cows at high and low risk for developing acidosis: feeding, ruminating, and lying behavior. J Dairy Sci 2009;92(10):5067–78.

23. Zhang K, Chang G, Xu T, et al. Lipopolysaccharide derived from the digestive tract activates inflammatory gene expression and inhibits casein synthesis in the mammary glands of lactating dairy cows. Oncotarget 2016;7(9):9652–65.

24. Bilal MS, Abaker JA, Ul Aabdin Z, et al. Lipopolysaccharide derived from the digestive tract triggers an inflammatory response in the uterus of mid-lactating dairy cows during SARA. BMC Vet Res 2016;12(1):284.

25. Wang YY, Li HP, Wang XJ, et al. Attenuated mRNA expression of lipid metabolism genes in primary hepatocytes following lipopolysaccharide treatment in dairy cows. Genet Mol Res 2015;14(2):3718–28.

26. Zebeli Q, Metzler-Zebeli BU, Ametaj BN. Meta-analysis reveals threshold level of rapidly fermentable dietary concentrate that triggers systemic inflammation in cattle. J Dairy Sci 2012;95(5):2662–72.

27. Gozho GN, Krause DO, Plaizier JC. Ruminal lipopolysaccharide concentration and inflammatory response during grain-induced subacute ruminal acidosis in dairy cows. J Dairy Sci 2007;90(2):856–66.

28. Rodriguez-Lecompte JC, Kroeker AD, Ceballos-Marquez A, et al. Evaluation of the systemic innate immune response and metabolic alterations of nonlactating cows with diet-induced subacute ruminal acidosis. J Dairy Sci 2014;97(12): 7777–87.

29. Eckersall PD, Young FJ, McComb C, et al. Acute phase proteins in serum and milk from dairy cows with clinical mastitis. Vet Rec 2001;148(2):35–41.

30. Hirvonen J, Huszenicza G, Kulcsar M, et al. Acute-phase response in dairy cows with acute postpartum metritis. Theriogenology 1999;51(6):1071–83.

31. Ahrens FA. Histamine, lactic acid, and hypertonicity as factors in the development of rumenitis in cattle. Am J Vet Res 1967;28(126):1335–42.

32. Underwood WJ. Rumen lactic acidosis: I. Epidemiology and pathophysiology. Compend Contin Educ Pract Vet 1992;14(8):1127–34.

33. Aschenbach JR, Oswald R, Gabel G. Transport, catabolism and release of histamine in the ruminal epithelium of sheep. Pflugers Arch 2000;440(1):171–8.

34. Shi Y, Weimer PJ. Response surface analysis of the effects of pH and dilution rate on Ruminococcus flavefaciens FD-1 in cellulose-fed continuous culture. Appl Environ Microbiol 1992;58(8):2583–91.

35. Krajcarski-Hunt H, Plaizier JC, Walton JP, et al. Short communication: effect of subacute ruminal acidosis on in situ fiber digestion in lactating dairy cows. J Dairy Sci 2002;85(3):570–3.

36. Griinari JM, Dwyer DA, McGuire MA, et al. Trans-octadecenoic acids and milk fat depression in lactating dairy cows. J Dairy Sci 1998;81(5):1251–61.

37. Gao X, Oba M. Relationship of severity of subacute ruminal acidosis to rumen fermentation, chewing activities, sorting behavior, and milk production in lactating dairy cows fed a high-grain diet. J Dairy Sci 2014;97(5):3006–16.

38. Graham C, Simmons NL. Functional organization of the bovine rumen epithelium. Am J Physiol Regul Integr Comp Physiol 2005;288(1):R173–81.

39. Steele MA, AlZahal O, Hook SE, et al. Ruminal acidosis and the rapid onset of ruminal parakeratosis in a mature dairy cow: a case report. Acta Vet Scand 2009;51:39.

40. Dirksen GU, Liebich HG, Mayer E. Adaptive changes of the ruminal mucosa and their functional and clinical significance. Bovine Pract 1985;20:116–20.

41. Krehbiel CR, Britton RA, Harmon DL, et al. The effects of ruminal acidosis on volatile fatty acid absorption and plasma activities of pancreatic enzymes in lambs. J Anim Sci 1995;73(10):3111–21.

42. Gressley TF, Hall MB, Armentano LE. Ruminant nutrition symposium: productivity, digestion, and health responses to hindgut acidosis in ruminants. J Anim Sci 2011;89(4):1120–30.

43. Li S, Khafipour E, Krause DO, et al. Effects of subacute ruminal acidosis challenges on fermentation and endotoxins in the rumen and hindgut of dairy cows. J Dairy Sci 2012;95(1):294–303.

44. Luan S, Cowles K, Murphy MR, et al. Effect of a grain challenge on ruminal, urine, and fecal pH, apparent total-tract starch digestibility, and milk composition of Holstein and Jersey cows. J Dairy Sci 2016;99(3):2190–200.

45. Nordlund KV, Cook NB, Oetzel GR. Investigation strategies for laminitis problem herds. J Dairy Sci 2004;87(E Suppl.):E27–35.

46. Argenzio RA, Henrikson CK, Liacos JA. Restitution of barrier and transport function of porcine colon after acute mucosal injury. Am J Physiol 1988;255(1 Pt 1): G62–71.

47. Golder HM, Denman SE, McSweeney C, et al. Ruminal bacterial community shifts in grain-, sugar-, and histidine-challenged dairy heifers. J Dairy Sci 2014;97(8): 5131–50.

48. Wetzels SU, Mann E, Pourazad P, et al. Epimural bacterial community structure in the rumen of Holstein cows with different responses to a long-term subacute ruminal acidosis diet challenge. J Dairy Sci 2016;100(3):1829–44.

49. Russell JB, Wilson DB. Why are ruminal cellulolytic bacteria unable to digest cellulose at low pH? J Dairy Sci 1996;79(8):1503–9.

50. Krause DO, Smith WJ, Conlan LL, et al. Diet influences the ecology of lactic acid bacteria and Escherichia coli along the digestive tract of cattle: neural networks and 16S rDNA. Microbiology 2003;149(Pt 1):57–65.

51. Russell JB, Rychlik JL. Factors that alter rumen microbial ecology. Science 2001; 292(5519):1119–22.

52. Rezac DJ, Thomson DU, Siemens MG, et al. A survey of gross pathologic conditions in cull cows at slaughter in the Great Lakes region of the United States. J Dairy Sci 2014;97(7):4227–35.

53. Bramley E, Costa ND, Fulkerson WJ, et al. Associations between body condition, rumen fill, diarrhoea and lameness and ruminal acidosis in Australian dairy herds. N Z Vet J 2013;61(6):323–9.

54. Nocek JE. Bovine acidosis: implications on laminitis. J Dairy Sci 1997;80(5): 1005–28.

55. Mungall BA, Kyaw-Tanner M, Pollitt CC. In vitro evidence for a bacterial pathogenesis of equine laminitis. Vet Microbiol 2001;79(3):209–23.

56. Danscher AM, Enemark JM, Telezhenko E, et al. Oligofructose overload induces lameness in cattle. J Dairy Sci 2009;92(2):607–16.

57. Kaur N, Gupta AK. Applications of inulin and oligofructose in health and nutrition. J Biosci 2002;27(7):703–14.

58. Kleen JL, Hooijer GA, Rehage J, et al. Subacute ruminal acidosis in Dutch dairy herds. Vet Rec 2009;164(22):681–3.

59. Zhang R, Huo W, Zhu W, et al. Characterization of bacterial community of raw milk from dairy cows during subacute ruminal acidosis challenge by high-throughput sequencing. J Sci Food Agric 2015;95(5):1072–9.

60. Duffield T, Plaizier JC, Fairfield A, et al. Comparison of techniques for measurement of rumen pH in lactating dairy cows. J Dairy Sci 2004;87(1):59–66.

61. Steiner S, Neidl A, Linhart N, et al. Randomised prospective study compares efficacy of five different stomach tubes for rumen fluid sampling in dairy cows. Vet Rec 2015;176(2):50.

62. Lodge-Ivey SL, Browne-Silva J, Horvath MB. Technical note: bacterial diversity and fermentation end products in rumen fluid samples collected via oral lavage or rumen cannula. J Anim Sci 2009;87(7):2333–7.

63. Shen JS, Chai Z, Song LJ, et al. Insertion depth of oral stomach tubes may affect the fermentation parameters of ruminal fluid collected in dairy cows. J Dairy Sci 2012;95(10):5978–84.

64. Nordlund KV, Garrett EF. Rumenocentesis: a technique for collecting rumen fluid for the diagnosis of subacute rumen acidosis in dairy herds. Bovine Pract 1994; 28(1):109–12.

65. Mialon MM, Deiss V, Andanson S, et al. An assessment of the impact of rumenocentesis on pain and stress in cattle and the effect of local anaesthesia. Vet J 2012;194(1):55–9.

66. Strabel D, Ewy A, Kaufmann T, et al. Rumenocentesis: a suitable technique for analysis of rumen juice pH in cattle? Schweiz Arch Tierheilkd 2007;149(7):301–6.

67. Neubauer V, Humer E, Kroger I, et al. Differences between pH of indwelling sensors and the pH of fluid and solid phase in the rumen of dairy cows fed varying concentrate levels. J Anim Physiol Anim Nutr (Berl) 2017. [EPub ahead of print].

68. Falk M, Munger A, Dohme-Meier F. Technical note: a comparison of reticular and ruminal pH monitored continuously with 2 measurement systems at different weeks of early lactation. J Dairy Sci 2016;99(3):1951–5.

69. Enjalbert F, Videau Y, Nicot MC, et al. Effects of induced subacute ruminal acidosis on milk fat content and milk fatty acid profile. J Anim Physiol Anim Nutr (Berl) 2008;92(3):284–91.

70. Colman E, Fokkink WB, Craninx M, et al. Effect of induction of subacute ruminal acidosis on milk fat profile and rumen parameters. J Dairy Sci 2010;93(10): 4759–73.

71. Maekawa M, Beauchemin KA, Christensen DA. Effect of concentrate level and feeding management on chewing activities, saliva production, and ruminal pH of lactating dairy cows. J Dairy Sci 2002;85(5):1165–75.

72. Mirmazhari-Anwar V, Sharifi K, Mirshahi A, et al. Transabdominal ultrasonography of the ruminal mucosa as a tool to diagnose subacute ruminal acidosis in adult dairy bulls: a pilot study. Vet Q 2013;33(3):139–47.

73. Penn State Extension. Estimating physically effective fiber with the Penn State Particle Separator. 2013. Available at: http://extension.psu.edu/animals/dairy/news/2013/estimating-physically-effective-fiber-with-the-penn-state-particle-separator. Accessed February 21, 2017.

74. Oetzel GR. Undertaking nutritional diagnostic investigations. Vet Clin North Am Food Anim Pract 2014;30(3):765–88.

75. Beauchemin KA, Farr BI, Rode LM, et al. Effects of alfalfa silage chop length and supplementary long hay on chewing and milk production of dairy cows. J Dairy Sci 1994;77(5):1326–39.

76. Devries TJ, Dohme F, Beauchemin KA. Repeated ruminal acidosis challenges in lactating dairy cows at high and low risk for developing acidosis: feed sorting. J Dairy Sci 2008;91(10):3958–67.

77. Iwaniuk ME, Erdman RA. Intake, milk production, ruminal, and feed efficiency responses to dietary cation-anion difference by lactating dairy cows. J Dairy Sci 2015;98(12):8973–85.

78. Krause KM, Dhuyvetter DV, Oetzel GR. Effect of a low-moisture buffer block on ruminal pH in lactating dairy cattle induced with subacute ruminal acidosis. J Dairy Sci 2009;92(1):352–64.

79. Keunen JE, Plaizier JC, Kyriazakis I, et al. Short communication: effects of subacute ruminal acidosis on free-choice intake of sodium bicarbonate in lactating dairy cows. J Dairy Sci 2003;86(3):954–7.

80. Reynolds CK, Durst B, Lupoli B, et al. Visceral tissue mass and rumen volume in dairy cows during the transition from late gestation to early lactation. J Dairy Sci 2004;87(4):961–71.

81. Fairfield AM, Plaizier JC, Duffield TF, et al. Effects of prepartum administration of a monensin controlled release capsule on rumen pH, feed intake, and milk production of transition dairy cows. J Dairy Sci 2007;90(2):937–45.

82. Andersen JB, Sehested J, Ingvartsen L. Effect of dry cow feeding strategy on rumen pH, concentration of volatile fatty acids and rumen epithelium development. Acta Agric Scand Sect A Anim Sci 1999;49(3):149–55.

83. Golder HM, Celi P, Rabiee AR, et al. Effects of feed additives on rumen and blood profiles during a starch and fructose challenge. J Dairy Sci 2014;97(2):985–1004.

84. Chibisa GE, Gorka P, Penner GB, et al. Effects of partial replacement of dietary starch from barley or corn with lactose on ruminal function, short-chain fatty acid absorption, nitrogen utilization, and production performance of dairy cows. J Dairy Sci 2015;98(4):2627–40.

85. AlZahal O, Dionissopoulos L, Laarman AH, et al. Active dry Saccharomyces cerevisiae can alleviate the effect of subacute ruminal acidosis in lactating dairy cows. J Dairy Sci 2014;97(12):7751–63.

86. Chaucheyras-Durand FW, Walker ND, Bach A. Effects of active dry yeasts on the rumen microbial ecosystem: past, present and future. Anim Feed Sci Tech 2008; 145:5–26.

87. Mutsvangwa T, Walton JP, Plaizier JC, et al. Effects of a monensin controlled-release capsule or premix on attenuation of subacute ruminal acidosis in dairy cows. J Dairy Sci 2002;85(12):3454–61.

88. Osborne JK, Mutsvangwa T, Alzahal O, et al. Effects of monensin on ruminal forage degradability and total tract diet digestibility in lactating dairy cows during grain-induced subacute ruminal acidosis. J Dairy Sci 2004;87(6):1840–7.

89. Martin SA. Manipulation of ruminal fermentation with organic acids: a review. J Anim Sci 1998;76(12):3123–32.

90. De Nardi R, Marchesini G, Plaizier JC, et al. Use of dicarboxylic acids and polyphenols to attenuate reticular pH drop and acute phase response in dairy heifers fed a high grain diet. BMC Vet Res 2014;10:277.

91. Balcells J, Aris A, Serrano A, et al. Effects of an extract of plant flavonoids (Bioflavex) on rumen fermentation and performance in heifers fed high-concentrate diets. J Anim Sci 2012;90(13):4975–84.

92. Calsamiglia S, Busquet M, Cardozo PW, et al. Invited review: essential oils as modifiers of rumen microbial fermentation. J Dairy Sci 2007;90(6):2580–95.

Diagnosis and Management of Rumen Acidosis and Bloat in Feedlots

Nathan F. Meyer, MS, MBA, PhD, DVM[a,b,*], Tony C. Bryant, MS, PhD[a,c]

KEYWORDS

- Acidosis • Bloat • Feedlot • Diagnosis • Rumen

KEY POINTS

- Ruminal bloat and ruminal acidosis represent the most common digestive disorders in feedlot cattle.
- Prevention of digestive disorders focuses on proper grain adaptation, sufficient ration fiber, ionophore inclusion, and minimizing feed variation.
- Diagnosis of digestive disorders should include a thorough feed and treatment history, evaluation of animals in their home environment, and complete necropsy.
- Treatment of digestive disorders depends on the specific digestive disorder and severity. A large number of animals may be affected so triage becomes critical to minimize impacts.
- Numerous animal and operational variables determine the digestive disorder prevalence, preventive techniques, treatment options, and overall impacts of digestive disorders in the feedlot.

INTRODUCTION

Most beef cattle in North America are raised on pasture for most their lives and then are finished in a feedlot on a high-concentrate diet composed of cereal grains such as corn, wheat, or barley. Economics favor a grain-finishing production system because of several factors, including reduced cost per unit of energy and resulting improved growth efficiencies associated with grains compared with roughages; availability of grains and land; logistical, storage, and operational efficiencies of transporting and handling grain; consistency of the nutrient profile of grains; and the quality and flavor aspects of beef produced from grain-fed cattle. The rumen is remarkably adaptable to

Disclosure: The authors have nothing to disclose.
[a] JBS Five Rivers Cattle Feeding, LLC, 1770 Promontory Circle, Greeley, CO 80634, USA; [b] Department of Clinical Sciences, Colorado State University, 1678 Campus Delivery, Fort Collins, CO 80523, USA; [c] Department of Animal Sciences, Colorado State University, 350 W Pitkin Street, Fort Collins, CO 80521, USA
* Corresponding author. 1770 Promontory Circle, Greeley, CO 80634.
E-mail address: Nathan.Meyer@jbssa.com

Vet Clin Food Anim 33 (2017) 481–498
http://dx.doi.org/10.1016/j.cvfa.2017.06.005
0749-0720/17/© 2017 Elsevier Inc. All rights reserved.

digest both forage and grain, and health challenges are common to cattle in each production phase. During the traditional feedlot phase of production, digestive disorders such as acidosis and bloat can result from the rapid fermentation of grain in the rumen. Understanding contributing causes and management factors that can help mitigate these potential maladies is important in order to optimize cattle production and health.

PREVALENCE OF DIGESTIVE-RELATED MORTALITY

Compared with other causes of mortality in the feedlot, digestive-related mortalities comprise 19.5% to 28.4% of all mortalities.[1–3] An internal database was examined that represented 4,487,364 head of cattle marketed between the years 2014 and 2016 in 11 feedlots ranging from southern Idaho to southern Arizona. In these feedlots and over this time frame, digestive mortality represented 0.073% (percentage of monthly occupancy) with a range from 0.064% (2016) to 0.082% (2015).[2] In addition, digestive mortality accounted for 26.9% of all mortalities with a range of 25.3% (2016) to 28.4% (2015). This prevalence was similar to that found by Vogel and Parrott,[3] who reported an average monthly digestive mortality of 0.06% (range, 0.05%–0.08%) and digestive mortality comprising 25.9% of all mortalities. In a more recent publication by Vogel and colleagues,[1] an analysis was performed from an industry feedlot database with closeout records from 2005 to 2014. This analysis revealed that 19.5% of mortalities were digestive related, with a range of 0.039% to 0.049% monthly digestive mortality, and the average day-on-feed at death was day 99. In addition, digestive mortality tends to be positively correlated with days on feed and with the beta-agonist feeding period.[1,4,5] Anecdotally, the investigators have observed that Holsteins and cattle housed in feed yards at higher elevations are more at risk of bloat. In addition, it has been observed that cattle in feedlots north of 38° north latitude have a higher prevalence of digestive mortality.[2] This finding could be a function of genetics, weather, or other factors associated with more northern latitudes.

An analysis of mortalities diagnosed as bloat or acidosis provides the relative contribution of each diagnosis to total digestive-related mortality.[2] From the years 2014 to 2015, 96.3% of all digestive mortalities were diagnosed as bloat compared with 3.7% diagnosed as acidosis. From a mortality standpoint, the contribution of bloat to digestive-related mortality represents most cases.

RUMINAL ACIDOSIS REVIEW

Ruminal acidosis in feedlot cattle can occur when rumen osmolality increases because of accumulation of lactate, short-chain fatty acids (ie, volatile fatty acids [VFAs]), and glucose. As a result, rumen pH decreases and the body reacts in a protective fashion by reducing feed intake and reducing acid absorption.[6,7] Lactate accumulation predominates in acute acidosis from the increased rate of production of glucose and reduced use of glucose, causing lactic acid–forming bacteria to proliferate.[8] The significance of ruminal lactate concentrations in subacute and acute acidosis seems to differ.[9] Researchers have indicated that concentration of total organic acids is of greater significance in subacute acidosis[10] and lactate may be of greater significance in acute acidosis.[11] As a result of ruminal acid accumulation, the ruminal osmotic pressure exceeds that of blood, resulting in a concentration gradient and a net flux of water into the rumen. This high osmotic pressure and influx of water can cause diarrhea and dehydration as well as damage to the rumen epithelium causing rumenitis (**Fig. 1**).[6]

During repair, the rumen wall can be thickened, and ruminal papillae can be altered, resulting in parakeratosis.[12] This resulting damage to the rumen epithelial wall can

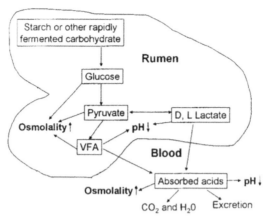

Fig. 1. The cause of acidosis in cattle. (*Adapted from* Owens FN, Secrist DS, Hill WJ, et al. Acidosis in cattle: a review. J Anim Sci 1998;76(1):277; with permission.)

increase permeability, which can have long-term effects on both nutrient and toxin absorption.[13,14] The rumen microbial population also changes with the changing rumen pH and with increased lactate accumulation so that lactate producers such as *Streptococcus bovis* and *Lactobacillus* spp proliferate and protozoa and cellulolytic microbes decline.[8,15–19] Entodiniomorph protozoa are known to engulf and sequester starch and ferment it at a slower rate than bacteria; however, the reduction of these ciliates during acidosis may provide for a less stable rumen environment.[18,20,21] The altered microbial composition, reduced salivation, and reduced ruminal pH can also decrease fiber digestibility, which can exacerbate the issue further.[17,22–24]

Endotoxins such as lipopolysaccharides and amines such as histamines can also be released from microbes because of the lysis of microbial cells that occurs at low pH, and these are then absorbed more easily across the damaged rumen wall.[14,19,25–28] These products, along with the damaged rumen epithelium, can affect rumen motility and can contribute to other ailments associated with acidosis, such as bloat, laminitis, liver abscesses, polioencephalomalacia, and death.[7,25,29] If the rumen pH cannot be equilibrated, the acids will be absorbed into the blood. Consequently, if the bicarbonate buffering capacity of the body is overwhelmed, systemic acidosis can result.

CLINICAL FINDINGS

Ruminal acidosis can vary from a mild indigestion to subacute acidosis to an acute and often fatal metabolic acidosis. When acidosis is suspected, a thorough history should be collected, including ration composition, milling records, and feed records. In addition, feed transition schedules and feed step-ups can aid in understanding the risk of ruminal acidosis. Severity of ruminal acidosis is a function of time below a specified threshold pH (5.2) and magnitude below the threshold. Animal variation also exists in tolerance to acidosis, as shown by intraruminally placed pH meters and challenge models.[30] In cases of mild or subacute ruminal acidosis, cattle may show signs of colic and anorexia, and loose stools are commonly present. When an entire group of animals is affected, it is common to see a reduction in feed intake, and, as the home pen surface is evaluated, stools will be seen across the surface that have a shiny appearance and are mostly liquid. In addition, cattle commonly have an abnormal amount of manure smeared across their hindquarters. Mild or subacute acidosis is commonly seen during ration transitions, weather alterations, and mild feeding errors.

In severe cases of ruminal acidosis, the first indication of a problem is often a large decrease in feed consumption noticed by the feed caller. In addition, pen checkers notice cattle showing clinical signs consistent with ruminal acidosis. Cattle may be recumbent, some may be staggering, and severe anorexia is present. Recumbent animals often lie with their heads tucked in their flanks, similar to parturient paresis. Further examination reveals an absence of ruminal contractions, diminished or absent palpebral reflexes, severe dehydration, and animals that are severely lethargic. A profuse and malodorous diarrhea develops and grain is typically present in the stools at an abnormal quantity from the increased rate of passage and decreased digestibility.

Postmortem examination at the time of death reveals severe dehydration (eye recession), copious amounts of fluid in the gastrointestinal tract, and a low ruminal pH (<5.0). The mucosa of the ruminal papillae is brown, friable, and easily detaches, revealing a diffuse and severe rumenitis (**Fig. 2**).[31] Ruminal contents have an increased proportion of fluid and undigested grain and a sour smell.

TREATMENT

Once a presumptive diagnosis of acidosis has been made, the current feed should be evaluated and bunk scooped or ration altered to prevent cases from progressing or new cases developing. Cattle that are recumbent have a guarded to poor prognosis. Severely compromised cattle should be humanely euthanized.

Standing cattle should be offered grass hay and water and monitored until they are stable. Systemic antimicrobials, nonsteroidal antiinflammatory drugs, thiamine, fluid support, and oral magnesium hydroxide are often beneficial to address the varying effects of the insult.[32] Limited research is available on stepping cattle back up to a

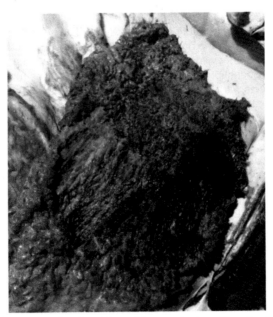

Fig. 2. Acute acidosis. Note the sloughing of the ruminal papillae revealing a diffuse and severe rumenitis.

finisher ration after an acidotic bout. It is common to wait a week after the initial insult and then begin a slow ration step-up program.

Laminitis, polioencephalomalacia, and liver abscesses are sequelae that can occur in cattle that recover from rumen acidosis. It is also the investigators' observation that cattle performance is severely affected following a severe acidosis insult and rarely does the animal or pen return to previous intake and performance. Salvage slaughter should be considered for cattle that do not respond to treatment or have a poor recovery.

RUMINAL BLOAT REVIEW

Bloat (ruminal tympany) results when excess gas accumulates in the rumen, resulting in increased intraruminal pressure and distention of the left dorsal abdominal wall, becoming apparent with protrusion of the paralumbar fossa area. Ruminal fermentation of feedstuffs by microbes generates gases, primarily carbon dioxide and methane. These gases are expelled from the rumen by absorption through the rumen wall, passage through to the next stomach compartment, or eructation through the esophagus; eructation through the esophagus is the predominant route for gas expulsion from the rumen.[33,34]

Eructation is a complex process involving integration of numerous organs by the central nervous system.[33] Ruminants use organ reticulorumen contractions to mix contents and for eructation. The primary contractions consist of 2 contractions of the reticulorumen fold and then a contraction that moves caudally. Eructation is associated with the secondary contractions and comprise contractions of the dorsal coronary pillar, caudodorsal blind sac, and dorsal sac, and relaxation of the caudoventral blind sac.[35] Contractions of the longitudinal and cranial pillars prevent digesta from filling the cranial sac and allows free gas in the dorsal sac to be expelled from the cardia. The multiple-stage eructation event is induced by increased ruminal gas and fill pressure, which is sensed by tension receptors located in the reticulum and cranial sac of the rumen.[35,36] The information from the tension receptors is transmitted via the afferent vagus nerve fibers to the central nervous system. If the distention is severe, then ruminal contractions are inhibited and result in ruminal atony.[37] During eructation, gas passes out of the rumen through the cardia into the esophagus and then pharynx. As the nasopharyngeal sphincter is closed, the gas is forced through the trachea and then into the lungs, where some gas is absorbed and the remainder exhaled.[33,36]

If the rate of gas production exceeds the rate of elimination, then bloat can result. In extreme situations, the increased gas accumulation and resulting ruminal distention can exert pressure on the diaphragm and lungs, which can inhibit respiration and may result in death by asphyxiation if not alleviated. Bloat can occur in cattle grazing pasture or in cattle housed in a feed yard and can occur in the forms of free-gas bloat or as frothy (foamy) bloat. Free-gas bloat usually results from one of the following causes: a physical obstruction (eg, potatoes, beets, hay twine) anterior to the rumen; damage to tissue such as the vagus nerve, cardia, or rumen; or changes in rumen motility.[34,36,38,39] Although not as common, free-gas bloat can also occur during lateral recumbency or be caused by hypocalcemia, acid indigestion, or esophageal stenosis from lesions, tumors, or inflammation.[36,40] If observed and diagnosed in a timely manner, free-gas bloat can typically be alleviated quickly by removing the obstruction from the esophagus or by intubating the rumen to expel the gas. In many cases, free-gas bloat arising from damaged tissue can become a chronic, recurring issue.

The predominant type of bloat in feedlot cattle is frothy bloat.[34,37] The rumen contents of feedlot cattle are normally stratified by the density of digesta, with the smaller and denser particles in the ventral rumen progressing dorsally to longer, less dense particles and then a gas layer in the dorsal sac that forms as gases produced by microbial activity rise as bubbles through the digesta.[41] Frothy bloat arises when a stable foam forms and then traps gases throughout the fluid phase of the rumen so that the digesta are less stratified.[38] The foam can be very persistent and can occupy the entire reticulorumen. The increased volume of rumen digesta can potentially impair the clearing of the cardia and inhibit eructation of gases.[33]

The formation of a stable foam is thought to be related to the release of excess stored mucopolysaccharides (or slime) from encapsulated rumen bacteria, release of other molecules including nucleic acids and carbohydrates during lysis of rumen microbial cells, and digestion of feedstuffs.[41–44] The increased quantity of nucleic acids and carbohydrate increases the viscosity of rumen fluid and is characteristic of feedlot bloat.[43–46] Saliva has been shown to have antifoaming characteristics.[47,48] Specifically, it was postulated that salivary mucin may be an antifoaming agent, and researchers showed that catabolism of mucin by mucinolytic bacteria was associated with bloat.[49] Consequently, decreased saliva production may be correlated to bloat occurrence.

Acidosis and bloat are interrelated disorders, and bouts of acidosis can predispose cattle to bloat. Ruminal contractions and motility are reduced by lactic acid, VFAs, endotoxins, and histamines, levels of which have been shown to increase during acidosis.[25] Some consequences of acidosis and increased rumen osmolality include decreased salivation, reduced rumen and intestinal motility and absorption, increased lysis of microbial cells, a change in the rumen microbiome, and decreased bacterial digestion of starch and fiber.[6,8,25] Altogether, rumen stasis and stagnation and reduced abomasal motility can cause gas to accumulate in the rumen and can lead to bloat.

CLINICAL FINDINGS

Primary ruminal bloat is one of the more straightforward diagnoses to make. In early stages of the disease, the left paralumbar fossa is mildly distended and abdominal distention is present. As bloat progresses and intraabdominal pressure increases, the distention in the left paralumbar fossa becomes more apparent, the rectum may protrude, and pressure on the diaphragm increases until the animal shows signs of respiratory distress, and a reluctance to move (**Fig. 3**).

In addition to clinical signs, other factors can aid in a presumptive diagnosis of bloat. In the feedlot, peak prevalence occurs at 99 to 120 days on feed,[1,2] and is seen most frequently during ration changes, weather alterations, and following variations in milling and feed delivery. During a bloat event, many of the factors that trigger bloat affect the entire group so it is common to see a range of clinical severities within in a group from mild to moderate abdominal distention to clinical bloat.[50]

A thorough individual and pen-level history should be collected at the time of death. In addition, noting the location and presentation of the animal at death and timely necropsy aid in an accurate diagnosis. Non–digestive-related causes of bloat mortality such as cast and a prolonged period from death to the time of necropsy may have identical postmortem lesions to bloat. A complete postmortem examination should be performed, examining all major organs and ruling out other causes of death.

Gross necropsy findings associated with bloat may include, but are not limited to, (1) congestion, hemorrhage, and edema of the anterior portion of the carcass, especially

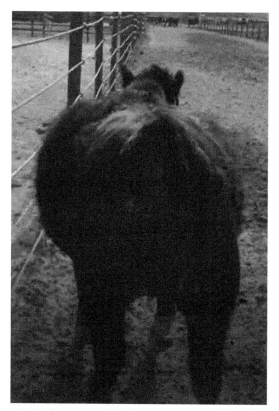

Fig. 3. Severe bloat. Note the severe distention in the area of the left paralumbar fossa.

in the area of the cervical muscles; (2) pallor of the semimembranosus and semitendinosus muscles of the hindquarters; (3) edema, often with emphysema between the muscles groups of the hindquarters, scrotum, and area of the mammary gland; (4) small and pale liver; (5) compressed lungs; and (6) presence of a tenacious froth or gas in the rumen.[50–52]

TREATMENT

Passage of a stomach tube is indicated for the initiation of the treatment of abdominal distention. The largest-bore tube of sufficient length to reach the dorsocaudal ruminal sac should be passed. Attempts should be made to clear the tube by blowing and the tube should be moved back and forth within the rumen to locate areas of gas that may be relieved.[50] If no gas is present, the tube should be removed and presence of froth within the tube should be examined. If the animal is not in respiratory distress or extremely colicky, surface-active agents such as mineral oil or dioctyl sodium sulfosuccinate may be administered.

Severely compromised animals require surgical intervention. A trocar and cannula in the left paralumbar fossa should be used to initiate immediate relief. With frothy bloat, a standard size instrument is often not sufficient, so a larger-bore (2.5-cm diameter) instrument or rumenotomy should be performed.[50] Salvage slaughter is a humane option for cattle that fail to respond to treatment and chronically bloat.

RUMINAL DIGESTION OF GRAINS AND FORAGES

Grains and forages are ingested, and the starch and fiber components within each feedstuff are digested by rumen microbes to form short-chain fatty acids (VFAs), including acetate, propionate, and butyrate. In addition, lactate and gases such as carbon dioxide, methane, hydrogen, nitrogen, oxygen, and hydrogen sulfide can be byproducts of ruminal digestion. The short-chain fatty acids are then absorbed through the rumen wall and are used by various tissues for production of glucose, fatty acids, and ketones. Grain processing methods such as steam flaking or rolling or grinding followed by fermentation, which results in high-moisture corn, are commonly used to help solubilize the protein matrix surrounding the starch molecules in the kernels, which then makes the starch more available to rumen microbial action, thereby increasing the efficiency of starch use. The cell wall components of forages such as cellulose and hemicellulose are digested more slowly than the starch in grains. This difference in the rate of digestion can potentially result in digestive and health challenges such as acidosis and bloat.

FACTORS AND MANAGEMENT CONSIDERATIONS AFFECTING ACIDOSIS AND BLOAT

A key challenge in management of digestive disorders is the acute to peracute nature of the disease resulting in failure to detect and treat in a timely manner. Records show a low level of detected morbidity attributed to bloat and acidosis compared with a high mortality.[2,31,53] The National Animal Health Monitoring System estimated that 71% of feed yards surveyed were affected by digestive problems, and the respondents only observed digestive-related issues in 4.2% of the cattle.[53]

Compared with other disease states, more than 500,000 treatment records were reviewed examining morbidity and mortality attributable to infectious pneumonia.[2] An average mortality/morbidity ratio of 3.79% was observed for cattle diagnosed with infectious pneumonia. Alternatively, when examining records of diseases attributable to bloat and acidosis, a different observation was made. For disease attributed to bloat and acidosis, an average mortality/morbidity ratio of 158.7% was observed. Clearly, focusing on prevention of digestive-related diseases is paramount to reducing overall mortality prevalence.

RATION TRANSITIONS

Digestive disorders such as acidosis and bloat are interrelated and are complex disease states. Before shipment to feed yards, most cattle are on a forage-based growing program. In a typical grazing scenario, intake is regulated predominantly by physical fill; however, on a high-concentrate diet, chemostatic regulation becomes the primary method of modulating intake.[6] Consequently, after arrival into a feed yard, cattle are normally transitioned slowly over a period of 3 or more weeks, starting with a diet of 45% to 55% concentrate and moving to an 85% to 95% concentrate diet in order for both the animal and the rumen microbial population to have ample time to adapt to diets containing readily fermentable carbohydrates.[54]

Cattle that are rapidly adapted to high-concentrate diets have more variable ruminal pH response, lower intakes, and increased incidence of acidosis.[55–57] If cattle are adjusted to diets up to 90% concentrate in less than 14 days, acidosis and poor performance can result.[54] In addition to time, managing energy intake level can be important for proper adaptation of cattle to high-concentrate diets, and many studies have shown that providing ad libitum intake during days 5 to 14 of the period of transition to high-concentrate diets usually results in dramatic reduction in intake.[54,58]

Consequently, a properly designed adaptation program for managing dietary changes and intake levels is an important aspect of transitioning cattle to diets containing high levels of readily fermentable carbohydrates.

BUNK MANAGEMENT

Although cattle are fed and managed as groups with multiple animals in a pen, large variation in intakes and rumen environments exists within a pen of cattle on any given day. Consequently, bunk management entails managing the bell curve of individuals within a pen of cattle by assessing cattle behavior, time at which all feed distributed in a bunk has been consumed, fecal consistency, and the health of the group. As a result, feed yard nutritionists tend to design feeding programs to find an optimal balance between productivity for most of the animals within the pen and trying to mitigate the risk of digestive disturbances for those cattle that are more susceptible to metabolic disorders. The capacity of animals to cope with grain and acid loads is highly variable, and on any given day animals within a pen are at different physiologic stages.[57] Animals that are more acid tolerant and that have the capability to adapt more quickly to dietary and ruminal changes likely consume more feed and are more productive.[54]

Many feed yards use a slick-bunk (or clean-bunk) feeding program in which the daily intake assignment for a pen is determined based on a bunk-scoring methodology that factors in assessments of cattle behavior, the amount of feed remaining in a bunk on a given day immediately before feeding, or the time at which cattle have consumed all the feed that was delivered to them on a given day. The goal of a slick-bunk feeding program is to maximize average intake over the feeding period while also minimizing the daily wastage of feed that can occur in an ad libitum feeding system. In a slick-bunk program, the feed yard and nutritionist strive to have most of the bunks on a feed yard void of feed immediately before the delivery of the subsequent day's feed allotment.

The challenges to managing a slick-bunk feeding program result from the daily variation that exists in the rumen environment, cattle behavior, pen conditions, weather changes, logistical hurdles that exist from milling and delivering feed each day, and ingredient and dietary composition. Consequently, alterations in any of these factors can result in a cascade of physiologic changes in the rumen that may predispose animals to digestive issues such as acidosis and bloat. Because most feed yards stock cattle in pens to provide 22 to 30 cm (9–12 inches) per animal, not all cattle can fit at the bunk at any one time.[59] Therefore, animals must spread their meals out throughout the day. In a feed yard setting, cattle tend to eat 8 to 12 meals per day, but there is large animal-to-animal variation as well as day-to-day variation in meal frequency and size.[60–63] Consequently, if there is a dramatic change in the proportion of animals that desire to consume feed at a given time, then the rate and quantity of feed consumed can increase dramatically, resulting in rapid changes in the rumen microbial and pH environments.[58] These engorgement and binge-eating events can be triggered by behavioral changes associated with weather and barometric pressure patterns or with variation in the time at which feed is delivered caused by logistical challenges. Therefore, social dominance structure and competition can be a factor in meal size and frequency and thereby affect the potential for digestive disorders.

The assignment of the pen's daily feed amount can have bearing on cattle behavior and meal patterns. Many feed yards use a methodical and objective feed-calling system to apply an intake assignment to a pen based on visual assessment of the bunks throughout the time period between when cattle are fed for the last time on one day and for the first time on the subsequent day; the objective of these bunk assessments is to determine when cattle completed eating all the feed delivered to their pen. Other programs are more subjective and rely on assessments of cattle behavior and of the proportion of animals in each pen that come to the bunk immediately after feed is delivered to the pen. In either case, if the intake assignment is drastically out of sync with the wants of the cattle, digestive disturbances can result. Nutritional programs are made even more complex with differences in cattle breeds, quality, age, and background; time of year; weather patterns; and changes in ingredient sources, moistures, and nutrient composition. If possible, the cattle populations that are more susceptible to bloat should be fed first in a sequence. Examples of these higher-risk populations may include Holsteins, cattle with more relative days on feed, and those on a beta-agonist. In order to minimize digestive upsets, a bunk management and nutritional program must strive for consistency in all aspects of intake assignment, ingredient quality, feed manufacturing, and feed delivery.

GRAIN TYPE AND PROCESSING

The grain type and degree of processing can also influence the rate and extent of digestion and hence the rumen environment and predisposition to digestive upsets. Grains vary in average starch content and are ranked in decreasing order as corn and sorghum (71%–76%), wheat (62%–65%), barley (57%–59%), and oats (44%).[64] Each grain type also has unique features related to the protein matrix that surrounds the starch; consequently, the rate and extent of ruminal degradation depend on the structure and type of the protein-starch matrix and the ability of rumen microbes to break down the starch within this matrix. In addition, several grain processing methods exist that can aid in this process. For example, the grain can be ground or dry-rolled, resulting in a smaller particle size and more surface area for microbes and enzymes to attack the starch. Grain can also be fermented into products such as high-moisture corn; this process breaks the pericarp, reduces particle size, and solubilizes the protein matrix that encompasses the starch molecules within the endosperm. Another common method of grain processing, steam flaking, entails gelatinizing the starch via application of steam and pressure. The total quantity and rate at which starch molecules are converted to ruminal short-chain fatty acids (VFAs), lactate, and gas are determined by the interaction of starch content, the grain processing method, and degree of processing. Taken altogether, these factors along with dietary inclusion levels of grain, roughage, and other ingredients can determine the risk to digestive upset. Therefore, it is difficult to assign the order of risk to grain type and processing method; however, because of their high starch content and rapid rate of ruminal fermentation, wheat and high-moisture corn can be feedstuffs that can elicit a rapid change in the rumen environment and a predisposition to acidosis or bloat in cattle. Similarly, although less ruminal fermentation occurs with steam-flaked corn than with wheat and high-moisture corn, a rapid fermentation rate can occur with steam-flaked corn that is processed to a higher degree. Total ruminal organic acid production is less with grains containing less starch and that are processed to a lesser degree; this results in a shift of starch digestion to the abomasum and small and large intestine for products like dry-rolled corn. However, dry-rolling of corn results in lower animal productivity and efficiency than products such as steam-flaked and high-moisture corn.[65] For example, recently it was shown that starches from whole, dry-rolled, high-moisture, and steam-flaked corn have ruminal disappearance rates of 75%, 70%, 91%, and 85%, respectively, and total tract disappearance of starch was 85%, 91%, 99%, and 99% for whole, dry-rolled, high-moisture, and steam-flaked corn, respectively. Consequently, a balance is sought between animal productivity and ruminal health; a slow rate of fermentation is better for prevention of acidosis, but a faster rate of degradation is better for energetic efficiency.[6] Assessments of degree of processing of grains include visual appraisal, particle size distribution, density, protein solubility, gas production, refractometry, enzymatic conversion of starch to glucose, and fecal starch content. For dry-rolled grains, the primary methods of quality assessment are visual appraisal and particle size distribution. Fermented products such as high-moisture corn are typically appraised for particle size distribution and protein solubility. The predominant methods for assessing the quality of steam-flaked corn are on-site bulk density and laboratory enzymatic starch availability, and most nutritionists target a starch availability of 52% to 71%.[66] Starch availability can be affected by moisture content and age of the grain, retention time in the steam chest, quantity of steam applied, roll settings, roll corrugation and wear, and storage of the grain after processing. As mentioned previously, as particle size decreases, more surface area is exposed to microbial enzymes; as a result, particle size of grain is negatively correlated to rate of digestion and viscosity or rumen contents.[34,67] Diets containing finely ground grain have also been associated with reduced salivation, increased gas production, and increased occurrence of bloat.[33,68] Grain type, variety, and degree of processing are important considerations for metabolic maladies such as bloat and acidosis and must be managed accordingly.

DIETARY FIBER

Although most feed yard diets are primarily composed of grain, numerous aspects of dietary forage play a critical role in ruminal and animal health and in minimizing risk for digestive upset. Roughage sources used in most feed yard diets have different physical and chemical profiles, which makes determining roughage value and equivalency difficult.[69] Numerous attempts to assess roughage quality have been made, but the most commonly used system of categorizing roughage components, the neutral detergent fiber (NDF) method, was devised by Van Soest,[70] in which forages are divided into a readily digestible fraction and an incompletely digestible fraction. Most feed yard nutritionists use NDF or acid detergent fiber (ADF) composition of forages for dietary formulation and roughage equivalency purposes. Before the NDF system, crude fiber content was commonly used; however, crude fiber underestimates the plant cell contents.[71] The NDF fraction is considered to be the incompletely digestible fraction of the feed and contains cellulose, hemicellulose, and lignin, whereas the ADF fraction contains cellulose and lignin. Dairy nutritionists further defined effective NDF (eNDF) on the ability of a feed to replace roughage in a diet so that the percentage of fat in milk produced by cows eating the ration is maintained.[72] The eNDF is based on particle size as well as adjustments for numerous other subjective factors; as a result, the eNDF values for feedstuffs is arbitrary.[64] Physically effective NDF (peNDF) is related to the physical characteristics of fiber, such as particle size, that stimulates chewing activity and establishes the biphasic stratification of ruminal contents with a pool of liquid and small particles sitting below a floating mat of large particles.[72] In the peNDF system of roughage comparison, long-grass hay is used as the reference feed and the peNDF of other forages are expressed as percentages (known as the physically effective factor) relative to long-grass hay, which is multiplied by the NDF content of the roughage. In high-roughage diets of dairy cows, particle size and peNDF have been positively correlated to increased chewing time, salivary output, and ruminal pH.[73–75] Although feedlot cattle chew and salivate less than cattle on increased forage diets, mixed results have been observed in correlating particle length of roughages and ruminal pH in feedlot cattle.[76,77] Limitations to the use of peNDF for dietary formulation also include reliance on book values for the physically effective factor, and this factor was generated from limited research data.[64] In addition, peNDF does not account for ruminal degradation of the roughage and may not be a good predictor of rumen pH.[64] Consequently, use of peNDF for dietary formulation purposes has not been widely adopted by feed yard nutritionists.[66] Despite the variable results associated with peNDF, most nutritionists strive for longer chop lengths on hay (75–125 mm [3–5 inches]) and silage (13–19 mm [0.5–0.75 inches]); however, longer chop lengths on corn silage result in more whole kernels and increased variation in particle size unless it is kernel processed.

In terms of dietary formulation, both source and concentration of roughage affect intakes of feedlot cattle. In addition, a recent review and analysis of published data revealed that dietary NDF and eNDF supplied by roughage account for 92% and 93%, respectively, of intake responses observed in feed yard cattle, whereas dietary dry matter inclusion of roughages only accounted for 70% of the intake variation associated with roughage source and level.[69] Many feed yard nutritionists formulate diets based on the NDF solely supplied by the dietary roughage sources (ie, forage NDF or roughage NDF). Forage NDF has been correlated to ruminal pH, which may partially explain the relationship observed between forage NDF and intake.[69,73] Clinicians must be cognizant of the extreme variation that can exist in NDF or ADF content of feeds caused by roughage source, variety, maturity, and growing and harvest conditions. In addition, the fiber content of a single roughage can vary between sources (ie, farmer to farmer) and then be combined into 1 roughage supply pile or pit. Consequently, monitoring and adjusting for changing fiber content of feeds on a daily basis is extremely challenging; as a result, nutritionists tend to formulate for the average and assess and adjust for fiber changes over time. Because of the low inclusion of roughage in most feedlot diets, maintaining a minimal level of roughage in order to maintain a healthy and sustainable rumen environment is very important. Because diets are manufactured on an as-fed basis, extreme changes in moisture content of roughages caused by weather events or suppliers can have substantial impacts on the fiber composition of the diet. For example, if a roughage becomes extremely wet, the fiber content of the diet becomes reduced because of dilution with water if diets are not adjusted for moisture content of those ingredients. Therefore, monitoring for swings in moisture content of roughages is a key action that feed yards can do to ensure that the roughage requirements of cattle are met and to avoid digestive disturbances. Similarly, preceding and during storm events, cattle intakes can change dramatically; moreover, cattle intakes often increase in anticipation of a weather front. Consequently, ensuring that cattle have ample feed supplied to them as well as sufficient roughage is important. Most feed yards use so-called storm diets that contain higher inclusions of roughage for this purpose. Cattle must then be transitioned slowly off these diets and back to the regular diets.

In recent years, with the increased production of ethanol and other corn-derived byproducts for human consumption and use, the abundance of corn byproducts for cattle feed has increased, and wet corn gluten feed and corn distillers' grains have become more common in feedlot diets. Because of the reduction in total dietary starch associated with the use of these byproducts in place of cereal grains, it has been hypothesized that these corn byproducts may thereby reduce the prevalence of acidosis in feedlot cattle. Some studies have shown that use of wet corn gluten feed increases ruminal pH or reduces variation in ruminal pH, but less conclusive results exist with the inclusion of distillers' grains.[78–81] Consequently, these byproducts may have positive effects on rumen environment but should not be used as a replacement for roughage or for mitigation of digestive maladies.

FEED ADDITIVES

Feed additives are also used as aids in productivity and ruminal health in feedlot cattle. Ionophores such as monensin have been used extensively and others, including lasalocid and laidlomycin, have been investigated and used commercially. Ionophores are a unique set of antibiotics that affect bacterial cellular membranes, thus inhibiting cellular growth and replication.[82] In general, monensin selectively inhibits grampositive bacteria because of the absence of a complex outer membrane. However, monensin is also a potent inhibitor of *Butyrivibrio fibrisolvens*, a gram negative bacterium.[83]

Researchers have shown that monensin decreases meal size and quantity and daily feed intake variation while increasing meal frequency.[84,85] As a result of the changes in meals and bacterial population, monensin can increase ruminal pH and moderate changes in pH.[85] The modes of action of laidlomycin and lasalocid are similar to monensin, but at currently approved feeding levels these compounds seem to have less profound effects on the ruminal levels and intake patterns.[7]

Regardless of the primary role of lactate in acidosis, a reduction in lactate production is beneficial in prevention of acute acidosis and improving feed efficiency. Primary lactate-producing bacteria isolated include *S bovis* and *Lactobacillus* spp, and inhibition of these bacteria has been beneficial in reducing in vitro lactate production.[86] Nagaraja and colleagues[11] experimentally induced lactic acidosis by ruminally infusing glucose or finely ground corn. Cattle treated with monensin had higher ruminal pH and lower concentrations of the D (−) and L (+) isomers of lactate for the glucose challenge but did not prevent lactic acidosis in the fine-ground corn challenge. Differences could have been attributable to the amount of carbohydrate infused in the rumen (fine-ground corn was greater). Burrin and Britton[10] observed an increase in ruminal lactate concentrations without a concurrent decrease in pH when cattle were fed monensin. These observations could be attributed to a subacute acidotic state and a low correlation between lactate concentration and ruminal pH during subacute acidosis.[10] In general, monensin is effective at inhibiting lactate-producing bacteria, especially in acute acidosis, but the role of lactate inhibition in performance response observed with monensin feeding remains elusive.

Bartley and colleagues[87] described the effects of monensin and lasalocid on feedlot bloat. Cattle bloated on a high-grain diet were tested with a dose of 1.32 mg/kg BW (body weight) of lasalocid or monensin with bloat being reduced by 92% and 64%, respectively. In addition, cattle dosed with 0.66 mg/kg BW lasalocid prevented bloat from developing in cattle fed high-grain diets.

Most other feed additives and ingredients that have been researched have had no or inconclusive effects. For example, the addition of sodium bicarbonate to feedlot diets has had mixed results.[88,89] The use of detergents such as poloxalene have been shown to reduce pasture bloat but have not been effective in feedlot diets.[33] The addition of high levels of salt to the diets of feedlot cattle has had mixed outcomes.[90,91] The addition of mineral oil to feed yard diets has been shown to reduce bloat, and addition of soybean oil increased bloat, whereas tallow was neutral.[92] Current research focused on rumen health and cattle productivity is centered on the use of direct-fed microbials and probiotics such as *Lactobacillus acidophilus* and *Megasphaera elsdenii* and yeast fermentation products.

SUMMARY

Cattle feeding has progressed to an efficient and sustainable production system that converts available feedstuffs into beef products that satisfy consumers' needs.

Prevention of digestive disorders such as ruminal acidosis and bloat is achievable through a whole-systems approach. Dietary adaptation to high-concentrate diets, bunk management, grain source and degree of processing, roughage source and level, and feed additives can all affect productivity, rumen health, and digestive disturbances in feedlot cattle. Although prevention is a cornerstone, treatment and management of animals that are affected should be thorough and focus on the welfare of the animals. Numerous research opportunities exist in prevention and treatment of digestive disorders, especially as feeding programs and management systems change and new technologies become available.

REFERENCES

1. Vogel GJ, Bokenkroger CD, Rutten-Ramos SC, et al. A retrospective evaluation of animal mortality in US feedlots: rate, timing, and cause of death. Bov Pract 2015; 49(2):113–23.
2. Meyer NF, Bryant TC. Internal review of feedlot management and health records. 2017.
3. Vogel GJ, Parrott C. Mortality survey in feedyards: the incidence of death from digestive, respiratory, and other causes in feedyards on the great plains. Compendium on Continuing Education for the Practicing Veterinarian 1994;16(2): 227–34.
4. Loneragan GH, Dargatz DA, Morley PS, et al. Trends in mortality ratios among cattle in US feedlots. J Am Vet Med Assoc 2001;219(8):1122–7.
5. Loneragan GH, Thomson DU, Scott HM. Increased mortality in groups of cattle administered the β-adrenergic agonists ractopamine hydrochloride and zilpaterol hydrochloride. PLoS One 2014;9(3):e91177.
6. Owens FN, Secrist DS, Hill WJ, et al. Acidosis in cattle: a review. J Anim Sci 1998; 76(1):275–86.
7. Galyean ML, Rivera JD. Nutritionally related disorders affecting feedlot cattle. Can J Anim Sci 2003;83(1):13–20.
8. Slyter LL. Influence of acidosis on rumen function. J Anim Sci 1976;43(4):910–29.
9. Harmon DL, Britton RA, Prior RL, et al. Net portal absorption of lactate and volatile fatty acids in steers experiencing glucose-induced acidosis or fed a 70% concentrate diet ad libitum. J Anim Sci 1985;60:560–9.
10. Burrin DG, Britton RA. Response to monensin in cattle during subacute acidosis. J Anim Sci 1986;63:888–93.
11. Nagaraja TG, Avery TB, Bartley EE, et al. Prevention of lactic acidosis in cattle by lasalocid or monensin. J Anim Sci 1981;53:206–16.
12. Ørskov ER. Starch digestion and utilization in ruminants. J Anim Sci 1986;63(5): 1624–33.
13. Krehbiel CR, Britton RA, Harmon DL, et al. The effects of ruminal acidosis on volatile fatty acid absorption and plasma activities of pancreatic enzymes in lambs. J Anim Sci 1995;73(10):3111–21.
14. Aschenbach JR, Gäbel G. Effect and absorption of histamine in sheep rumen: significance of acidotic epithelial damage. J Anim Sci 2000;78(2):464–70.
15. Hungate RE, Dougherty RW, Bryant MP, et al. Microbiological and physiological changes associated with acute indigestion in sheep. Cornell Vet 1952;42:423–47.
16. Elam CJ. Acidosis in feedlot cattle: practical observations. J Anim Sci 1976;43(4): 898–901.
17. Russell JB, Wilson DB. Why are ruminal cellulolytic bacteria unable to digest cellulose at low pH? J Dairy Sci 1996;79(8):1503–9.

18. Goad DW, Goad CL, Nagaraja TG. Ruminal microbial and fermentative changes associated with experimentally induced subacute acidosis in steers. J Anim Sci 1998;76(1):234–41.
19. Nagaraja TG, Titgemeyer EC. Ruminal acidosis in beef cattle: the current microbiological and nutritional outlook. J Dairy Sci 2007;90(Suppl 1):E17–38.
20. Mackie RI, Gilchrist FMC. Changes in lactate-producing and lactate-utilizing bacteria in relation to pH in the rumen of sheep during stepwise adaptation to a high-concentrate diet. Appl Environ Microbiol 1979;38(3):422–30.
21. Bonhomme A. Rumen ciliates: their metabolism and relationships with bacteria and their hosts. Anim Feed Sci Technology 1990;30(3–4):203–66.
22. Burroughs W, Gerlaugh P, Edgington BH, et al. The influence of corn starch upon roughage digestion in cattle. J Anim Sci 1949;8(2):271–8.
23. Mould FL, Ørskov ER. Manipulation of rumen fluid pH and its influence on cellulolysis in sacco, dry matter degradation and the rumen microflora of sheep offered either hay or concentrate. Anim Feed Sci Technology 1983;10(1):1–14.
24. Calsamiglia S, Ferret A, Devant M. Effects of pH and pH fluctuations on microbial fermentation and nutrient flow from a dual-flow continuous culture system. J Dairy Sci 2002;85(3):574–9.
25. Huber TL. Physiological effects of acidosis on feedlot cattle. J Anim Sci 1976; 43(4):902–9.
26. Nagaraja TG, Bartley EE, Fina LR, et al. Evidence of endotoxins in the rumen bacteria of cattle fed hay or grain. J Anim Sci 1978;47(1):226–34.
27. Russell JB. Strategies that ruminal bacteria use to handle excess carbohydrate. J Anim Sci 1998;76(7):1955–63.
28. Gozho GN, Krause DO, Plaizier JC. Ruminal lipopolysaccharide concentration and inflammatory response during grain-induced subacute ruminal acidosis in dairy cows. J Dairy Sci 2007;90(2):856–66.
29. Brent BE. Relationship of acidosis to other feedlot ailments. J Anim Sci 1976; 43(4):930–5.
30. Cooper RJ, Klopfenstein TJ, Stock RA, et al. Observations on acidosis through continual feed intake and ruminal pH monitoring. Nebraska beef report. Lincoln (NE): University of Nebraska; 1998. p. 75–6. Available at: http://digitalcommons.unl.edu/animalscinbcr/329/.
31. Gelberg HB. Alimentary system. In: McGavin MD, Zachary JF, editors. Pathologic basis of veterinary disease. 4th edition. St Louis (MO): Mosby; 2007. p. 326–30.
32. Constable PD, Lorenz I. Grain overload in ruminants. In: Merck veterinary manual. 2016. Available at: http://www.merckvetmanual.com/digestive-system/diseases-of-the-ruminant-forestomach/grain-overload-in-ruminants. Accessed January 28, 2017.
33. Clarke RT, Reid CS. Foamy bloat of cattle. A review. J Dairy Sci 1974;57(7): 753–85.
34. Cheng KJ, McAllister TA, Popp JD, et al. A review of bloat in feedlot cattle. J Anim Sci 1998;76(1):299–308.
35. Krehbiel CR. Invited review: applied nutrition of ruminants: fermentation and digestive physiology. Prof Anim Scientist 2014;30(2):129–39.
36. Garry F. Managing bloat in cattle. Vet Med 1990;643–50.
37. Howarth RE, Chaplin RK, Cheng KJ, et al. Bloat in cattle, vol. 1858/E. Ontario (Canada): Agriculture Canada Publication; 1991. p. 1–32.
38. Howarth RE. A review of bloat in cattle. Can Vet J 1975;16(10):281–94.
39. Vasconcelos JT, Galyean ML. ASAS centennial paper: contributions in the journal of animal science to understanding cattle metabolic and digestive disorders. J Anim Sci 2008;86(7):1711–21.

40. Nagaraja TG. Bloat in feedlot cattle. Paper presented at: Cattle Drive '94 — A Canadian Feedlot Health and Nutrition Symposium. Kansas Agricultural Experiment Station. Manhattan (KS): University Extension Publication; 1994. p. 1–16.

41. Hungate RE, Fletcher DW, Dougherty RW, et al. Microbial activity in the bovine rumen: its measurement and relation to bloat. Appl Microbiol 1955;3(3):161–73.

42. Gutierrez J, Davis RE, Lindahl IL, et al. Bacterial changes in the rumen during the onset of feed-lot bloat of cattle and characteristics of *Peptostreptococcus elsdenii* n. sp. Appl Microbiol 1959;7(1):16–22.

43. Gutierrez J, Davis RE, Lindahl IL. Some chemical and physical properties of a slime from the rumen of cattle. Appl Microbiol 1961;9(3):209–12.

44. Cheng KJ, Hironaka R, Jones GA, et al. Frothy feedlot bloat in cattle: production of extracellular polysaccharides and development of viscosity in cultures of *Streptococcus bovis*. Can J Microbiol 1976;22(4):450–9.

45. Jacobson DR, Lindahl IL, McNeill JJ, et al. Feedlot bloat studies. II. Physical factors involved in the etiology of frothy bloat. J Anim Sci 1957;16(2):515–24.

46. Gutierrez J, Essig HW, Williams PP, et al. Properties of a slime isolated from the rumen fluid of cattle bloating on clover pasture. J Anim Sci 1963;22(2):506–9.

47. Bartley EE, Yadava IS. Bloat in cattle. IV. The role of bovine saliva, plant mucilages, and animal mucins. J Anim Sci 1961;20(3):648–53.

48. Van Horn HH, Bartley EE. Bloat in cattle. I. Effect of bovine saliva and plant mucin on frothing rumen contents in alfalfa bloat. J Anim Sci 1961;20(1):85–7.

49. Mishra BD, Fina LR, Bartley EE, et al. Bloat in cattle. XI. The role of rumen aerobic (facultative) mucinolytic bacteria. J Anim Sci 1967;26(3):606–12.

50. Constable PD, Lorenz I. Bloat in ruminants. In: Merck veterinary manual. 2016. Available at: http://www.merckvetmanual.com/digestive-system/diseases-of-the-ruminant-forestomach/bloat-in-ruminants. Accessed January 28, 2017.

51. Guard CL, Fecteau G. Frothy bloat. In: Smith BP, editor. Large animal internal medicine. 4th edition. St Louis (MO): Elsevier; 2009. p. 855–7.

52. Miles DG, Hoffman BW, Rogers KC, et al. Diagnosis of digestive deaths. J Anim Sci 1998;76:320–2.

53. USDA. Feedlot 2011. Part II: trends in health and management practices on U.S. feedlots, 1994-2011. National Animal Health Monitoring System. 2013. Available at: https://www.aphis.usda.gov/aphis/ourfocus/animalhealth/monitoring-and-surveillance/nahms/nahms_feedlot_studies.

54. Brown MS, Ponce CH, Pulikanti R. Adaptation of beef cattle to high-concentrate diets: performance and ruminal metabolism. J Anim Sci 2006;84(13_Suppl):E25–33.

55. Burrin DG, Stock RA, Britton RA. Monensin level during grain adaption and finishing performance in cattle. J Anim Sci 1988;66(2):513–21.

56. Brown MS, Krehbiel CR, Duff GC, et al. Effect of degree of corn processing on urinary nitrogen composition, serum metabolite and insulin profiles, and performance by finishing steers. J Anim Sci 2000;78(9):2464–74.

57. Bevans DW, Beauchemin KA, Schwartzkopf-Genswein KS, et al. Effect of rapid or gradual grain adaptation on subacute acidosis and feed intake by feedlot cattle. J Anim Sci 2005;83(5):1116–32.

58. Schwartzkopf-Genswein KS, Beauchemin KA, Gibb DJ, et al. Effect of bunk management on feeding behavior, ruminal acidosis and performance of feedlot cattle: a review. J Anim Sci 2003;81(14_suppl_2):E149–58.

59. Simroth JC, Thomson DU, Schwandt EF, et al. A survey to describe current cattle feedlot facilities in the High Plains region of the United States. Prof Anim Scientist 2017;33(1):37–53.

60. Gibb DJ, McAllister TA, Huisma C, et al. Bunk attendance of feedlot cattle monitored with radio frequency technology. Can J Anim Sci 1998;78(4):707–10.

61. Buhman MJ, Perino LJ, Galyean ML, et al. Eating and drinking behaviors of newly received feedlot calves. Prof Anim Scientist 2000;16(4):241–6.

62. Parsons CH, Galyean ML, Swingle RS, et al. Use of individual feeding behavior patterns to classify beef steers into overall finishing performance and carcass characteristic categories. Prof Anim Scientist 2004;20(4):365–71.

63. Schwartzkopf-Genswein KS, Beauchemin KA, McAllister TA, et al. Effect of feed delivery fluctuations and feeding time on ruminal acidosis, growth performance, and feeding behavior of feedlot cattle. J Anim Sci 2004;82(11):3357–65.

64. NRC. Nutrient requirements of beef cattle. 8th revised edition. Washington, DC: Natl Acad Press; 2016.

65. Owens FN, Secrist DS, Hill WJ, et al. The effect of grain source and grain processing on performance of feedlot cattle: a review. J Anim Sci 1997;75(3):868–79.

66. Vasconcelos JT, Galyean ML. Nutritional recommendations of feedlot consulting nutritionists: the 2007 Texas Tech University survey. J Anim Sci 2007;85(10):2772–81.

67. Richards CJ, Hicks B. Processing of corn and sorghum for feedlot cattle. Vet Clin North Am Food Anim Pract 2007;23(2):207–21.

68. Hironaka R, Miltimore JE, McArthur JM, et al. Influence of particle size of concentrate on rumen conditions associated with feedlot bloat. Can J Anim Sci 1973;53(1):75–80.

69. Galyean ML, Defoor PJ. Effects of roughage source and level on intake by feedlot cattle. J Anim Sci 2003;81(14_suppl_2):E8–16.

70. Van Soest PJ. Development of a comprehensive system of feed analyses and its application to forages. J Anim Sci 1967;26(1):119–28.

71. Jung HJ. Analysis of forage fiber and cell walls in ruminant nutrition. J Nutr 1997;127(5):810S–3S.

72. Mertens DR. Creating a system for meeting the fiber requirements of dairy cows. J Dairy Sci 1997;80(7):1463–81.

73. Allen MS. Relationship between fermentation acid production in the rumen and the requirement for physically effective fiber. J Dairy Sci 1997;80(7):1447–62.

74. Yang WZ, Beauchemin KA. Increasing the physically effective fiber content of dairy cow diets may lower efficiency of feed use. J Dairy Sci 2006;89(7):2694–704.

75. Beauchemin KA, Eriksen L, Nørgaard P, et al. Short communication: salivary secretion during meals in lactating dairy cattle. J Dairy Sci 2008;91(5):2077–81.

76. Pitt RE, Van Kessel JS, Fox DG, et al. Prediction of ruminal volatile fatty acids and pH within the net carbohydrate and protein system. J Anim Sci 1996;74(1):226–44.

77. Nocek JE. Bovine acidosis: implications on laminitis. J Dairy Sci 1997;80(5):1005–28.

78. Krehbiel CR, Stock RA, Herold DW, et al. Feeding wet corn gluten feed to reduce subacute acidosis in cattle. J Anim Sci 1995;73(10):2931–9.

79. Sindt JJ, Drouillard JS, Thippareddi H, et al. Evaluation of finishing performance, carcass characteristics, acid-resistant *E. coli* and total coliforms from steers fed combinations of wet corn gluten feed and steam-flaked corn. J Anim Sci 2002;80(12):3328–35.

80. Montgomery SP, Drouillard JS, Titgemeyer EC, et al. Effects of wet corn gluten feed and intake level on diet digestibility and ruminal passage rate in steers. J Anim Sci 2004;82(12):3526–36.

81. Galyean ML, Hubbert ME. Traditonal and alternative sources of fiber - roughage values, effectiveness, and concentrations in starting and finishing diets. Paper presented at: Plains Nutrition Council 2012; San Antonio, TX, April 12-13, 2012.

82. Russell JB, Houlihan AJ. Ionophore resistance of ruminal bacteria and its potential impact on human health. FEMS Microbiol Rev 2003;27:65–74.

83. Bergen WG, Bates DB. Ionophores: their effect on production efficiency and mode of action. J Anim Sci 1984;58:1465–83.

84. Stock RA, Laudert SB, Stroup WW, et al. Effect of monensin and monensin and tylosin combination on feed intake variation of feedlot steers. J Anim Sci 1995; 73(1):39–44.

85. Erickson GE, Milton CT, Fanning KC. Interaction between bunk management and monensin concentration on finishing performance, feeding behavior, and ruminal metabolism during an acidosis challenge with feedlot cattle. J Anim Sci 2003; 81(11):2869–79.

86. Dennis SM, Nagaraja TG, Bartley EE. Effects of lasalocid or monensin on lactate-producing or -using rumen bacteria. J Anim Sci 1981;52:418–26.

87. Bartley EE, Nagaraja TG, Pressman ES, et al. Effects of lasalocid or monensin on legume or grain (feedlot) bloat. J Anim Sci 1983;56(6):1400–6.

88. Zinn RA. Comparative feeding value of steam-flaked corn and sorghum in finishing diets supplemented with or without sodium bicarbonate. J Anim Sci 1991; 69(3):905–16.

89. González LA, Ferret A, Manteca X, et al. Increasing sodium bicarbonate level in high-concentrate diets for heifers. I. Effects on intake, water consumption and ruminal fermentation. Animal 2008;2(5):705–12.

90. Elam CJ, Davis RE. Ruminal characteristics and bloat incidence in cattle as influenced by feeding synthetic saliva salts and sodium chloride. J Anim Sci 1962; 21(2):327–30.

91. Cheng KJ, Bailey CB, Hironaka R, et al. Bloat in feedlot cattle: effects on rumen function of adding 4% sodium chloride to a concentrate diet. Can J Anim Sci 1979;59(4):737–47.

92. Elam CJ, Davis RE. Ruminal characteristics and feedlot bloat incidence in cattle as influenced by vegetable oil, mineral oil, and animal fat. J Anim Sci 1962;21(3): 568–74.

Disorders of Rumen Distension and Dysmotility

Derek Foster, DVM, PhD

KEYWORDS

- Vagal indigestion • Rumen motility • Abdominal distension

KEY POINTS

- Rumen distension and hypomotility are common clinical signs that are found together.
- The location of abdominal distension and consistency of rumen contents provide key information for determining the cause of abdominal distension.
- Serum chloride and bicarbonate concentrations and rumen chloride concentration allow for differentiation of type 2 and type 3 vagal indigestion.
- Rumenotomy or right flank exploratory surgery can be both diagnostic and therapeutic.

INTRODUCTION

Rumen distension and dysmotility are not uncommon presentations in both cattle and small ruminants. These clinical signs often are linked, as dysmotility can lead to rumen distension and distension can lead to dysmotility. Identifying the underlying cause of the distension and dysmotility and determining if it is truly of gastrointestinal origin is critical to appropriate treatment. Generally, a thorough physical examination combined with some routine diagnostics can accurately identify the reason for rumen dysfunction, and guide appropriate treatment and prognosis.

NORMAL RUMEN CONTOUR AND MOTILITY

Examination of rumen shape, fill, and motility should be a part of the physical examination on all ruminants. Assessment of abdominal shape and rumen fill provides crucial information on feed intake and potential causes of distension. Decreased rumen motility can be a sensitive indicator of disease, although not specific, as many inflammatory processes and increased sympathetic tone will decrease normal rumen motility.[1]

Abdominal and Rumen Contour

Assessment of abdominal shape is preferably done early in a physical examination while observing a cow from a distance. While standing directly behind the cow,

Disclosure Statement: The author has nothing to disclose.
Department of Population Health and Pathobiology, NC State College of Veterinary Medicine, 1060 William Moore Drive, Raleigh, NC 27606, USA
E-mail address: derek_foster@ncsu.edu

http://dx.doi.org/10.1016/j.cvfa.2017.06.006
0749-0720/17/© 2017 Elsevier Inc. All rights reserved.
vetfood.theclinics.com

determine if the cow's abdomen appears gaunt, normal, or distended.[2] Abdominal shape is not entirely dictated by rumen shape, but rumen size is the most common reason for abnormal distension.[3] Abnormalities identified at this time can be useful in guiding a more thorough examination of the forestomach during the remainder of the physical examination. Nonetheless, practitioners must remember that other conditions, including intestinal distension, peritoneal effusion, pathologic accumulation of uterine fluid, and rupture of the prepubic tendon can affect abdominal shape and must be considered.

In a normal cow or small ruminant, the abdomen should be slightly wider than the stifles bilaterally. Typically, it will be somewhat symmetric, although slight differences from right to left are not uncommon. The most prominent distension on the left in a normal cow is typically around the level of the stifle in the mid abdomen due to fiber accumulation in the rumen. On the right, the normal shape is a slight enlargement below the stifle due to the small intestine.

The rumen should be palpated in the left paralumbar fossa and rectally. The normal rumen stratification can be identified on physical examination. There should be a gas cap in the caudodorsal rumen, a fiber mat throughout most of the rumen, and fluid ventrally. The gas cap, found dorsally, is softer and will immediately return to its previous shape when compressed. The doughy fiber mat is the most easily distinguished layer on palpation, as one can press into the rumen wall and leave an indention when it is palpated rectally. On palpation through the flank, the fiber mat simply feels firm. The fluid layer is found in the ventral left flank. This area is softer than the fiber mat, but ballottement of this area is difficult due to the weight of the rumen contents.

Normal Rumen Motility

Rumen motility should similarly be evaluated as a part of the physical examination of all ruminants. Simultaneous auscultation and palpation in the left paralumbar fossa will allow the examiner to assess the frequency and strength of rumen contractions while also hearing any abnormal sounds associated with the contraction. The normal rate is 1 to 3 contractions per 2 minutes. Each contraction should be strong enough to lift the examiner's hand on the paralumbar fossa. The sound should grow louder and then softer as the fiber mat turns inside the rumen and brushes along the rumen wall. There should not be any splashes or bubbling sounds associated with the contraction.[2] This assessment of rumen motility measures the contraction rate of the dorsal rumen sac, and does not differentiate primary versus secondary contraction, as the dorsal sac will contract with both patterns. In most cases, simply determining the overall rumen contraction rate is adequate.

Primary contractions are mixing contractions in which the fiber mat is turned in the rumen to ensure that feed material is mixed with the microbial flora contained in the rumen fluid. These contractions occur approximately 1 to 2 times per 2 minutes. Primary contractions are initiated at the reticulum with a biphasic contraction of the reticulum. These contractions can be ausculted at the seventh to eighth intercostal space, just caudal to the elbow on the left side or visualized by ultrasound caudal to the xiphoid and left of midline. The first reticular contraction is smaller, whereas the second contraction completely collapses the reticular lumen. From there, the contraction moves caudally and dorsally as the dorsal sac contracts. This is followed by contraction of the ventral sac and finally by contraction of the cranial sac to complete the cycle.[1,4] This pattern effectively mixes the fiber suspended in the mat with the liquid in the ventral aspect of the rumen, allowing the bacteria to attach to the undigested fiber. This furthers digestion and increases fermentation. Primary contractions also cause fluid outflow through the omasal canal as the reticular contractions create negative pressure in the canal causing fluid and fine feed material to be aspirated through the omasal orifice.[5]

Primary rumen contractions are controlled centrally at the dorsal vagal nucleus in the brainstem. Afferent fibers travel via the vagus nerve to the forestomach and allow for coordinated, regular primary contractions. Without this control, contractions become uncoordinated and insufficient to provide adequate mixing or allow for the removal of fluid and feed material from the rumen.[1] Normally the rumen has 1 to 2 primary contractions per 2 minutes.[6] Moderate rumen distension, as would be found after a recent meal, increases primary contraction rate due to stimulation of stretch receptors in the rumen wall, whereas severe pathologic distension will stop rumen contractions.[7] Abomasal distension will also reduce primary contractions, presumably to decrease the flow of ingesta through the omasal canal into the already overfull abomasum. Stimulation of buccal receptors in the mouth during feeding will also increase contraction rate, while chemoreceptors in the rumen epithelium monitor pH, and will stop rumen contractions if the pH drops below 5.0. Additional inhibitors of primary contractions are systemic disease and increased sympathetic tone (eg, pain, fear).[1]

Secondary contractions are defined as those that cause eructation, although this distinction is less clear in reality, as ruminants can eructate with primary contractions and do not always eructate with each secondary contraction. Further, secondary contractions have been defined differently by various researchers. Some view them as a standalone motility pattern,[8] whereas others have described them as an additional contraction cycle superimposed on a primary, mixing contraction.[4] Again, a strict definition here is likely inaccurate, as it appears that these patterns are not nearly as fixed as one would like, as different methods of recording contractions and species differences (sheep vs cattle) further muddy the characterization of contraction patterns.[9] Nonetheless, secondary contractions typically involve a contraction of the cranial pillar that holds ingesta back in the caudal sac, while a wave of contraction moves cranially across the dorsal sac, which pushes the gas cap forward.[10] This clears the cardia of fluid, which allows it to open, leading to eructation.

Secondary contractions typically occur following every other primary contraction, leading to 1 secondary contraction every 2 minutes.[6] Assessment of secondary contractions can be done by simultaneously listening to the reticulum and feeling rumen contractions in the left flank. As mentioned previously, primary contractions are felt immediately after a reticular contraction. Secondary contractions will be felt without an associated reticular contraction. The primary driver of secondary contractions is the rate of gas production and subsequent distension of the dorsal sac of the rumen.[10] Inhibition of secondary contractions is due to excessive distension and sympathetic tone. Eructation can be prevented even if the motility pattern is normal if the cardia is not able to be cleared of fluid.[11] This can occur if the animal is laterally recumbent or there is froth in the rumen.[12] Damage to the epithelium near the cardia from rumenitis can inhibit the ability of the cardia to sense the presence of gas, and subsequently prevent it from opening.

PHYSICAL EXAMINATION
Abnormal Rumen Contour and Motility

Abnormal abdominal and rumen shape
Finding that the cow's abdomen is narrower than her stifles suggests prolonged anorexia, as completely emptying the rumen can take several days. Although specific in identifying a significant and prolonged decrease in feed intake, a gaunt abdomen provides little guidance as to the underlying problem.[2]

If a cow is found to have a distended abdomen, first characterize the location of the distension, the organ leading to abdominal distension, and determine if the distension is due to the accumulation of gas, fluid, or feed material. The distension is most commonly found in the mid abdomen and dorsally on the left, ventrally on the right, dorsally on the left and ventrally on the right, or ventrally bilaterally. Other locations (ie, just ventrally on the left or just dorsally on the right) are less common due to the abdominal anatomy of ruminants.[3]

Once the distension is localized, ballottement of the abdomen and rectal palpation can be used to determine the organ or organs leading the change in abdominal shape and whether the abnormal distension is due to gas, fluid, or feed material. Based on the location and type of distension, the veterinarian can then develop a relatively short differential diagnosis list (**Table 1**).

Unilateral distension on the left side is almost always due to enlargement of the rumen. Palpation of the rumen at paralumbar fossa and rectally will allow practitioners to determine the reason for the distension. Excessive gas will accumulate dorsally, and will feel like a large balloon (**Fig. 1**). This is consistent with a type 1 vagal indigestion (failure of eructation). Excessive fluid distension of the left side is consistent with a rumen acidosis and the subsequent fluid shifts that occur due to osmosis. Early type 2 vagal indigestion (failure of rumen outflow) cases may have fluid distension only on the left, but most commonly they are distended bilaterally. An enlarged, doughy rumen is consistent with a feed impaction due to poor-quality feedstuffs or inactivity of the rumen microorganisms. Additional information on these disorders is provided later in this article and elsewhere in this issue.

Distension ventrally on the right side is most commonly either fluid or feed. If the distension is due to fluid, the most likely reasons are type 3 (failure of abomasal outflow) or 4 (failure of pyloric outflow) vagal indigestion or small intestinal distension. With type 3 or 4 vagal indigestion, the abomasum initially becomes distended and then, ultimately, the rumen becomes distended as well. Therefore, most of the animals present with bilateral distension. Cattle with small intestinal distension, on the other hand, may not have rumen distension, as they often present with signs of abdominal pain due to the stretch of the intestinal wall earlier in the disease process. Feed distension on the lower right side is consistent with an abomasal impaction.

Bilateral distension most commonly occurs due to fluid accumulation in the rumen or rumen and abomasum (**Fig. 2**). As fluid is trapped in the rumen, it initially distends on the left in the midflank. Over time, the ventral sac of the rumen expands greatly toward the right such that there is now distension of both sides. If there is a type 3 vagal indigestion, distension of the abomasum will contribute to the ventral, right-sided distension, and eventually fluid will back up into the rumen and cause the left-sided

Table 1
Locations and types of distension

Type of Distension	Dorsal Left	Ventral Right	Dorsal Left and Ventral Right	Ventral Bilaterally
Gas distension	Type 1 vagal indigestion	Uncommon	Uncommon	Uncommon
Fluid distension	Rumen acidosis	Type 3 or 4 vagal indigestion, small intestinal distension	Type 2 or 3 vagal indigestion	Peritoneal effusion, hydrops conditions
Feed material	Rumen impaction	Abomasal impaction	Uncommon	Uncommon

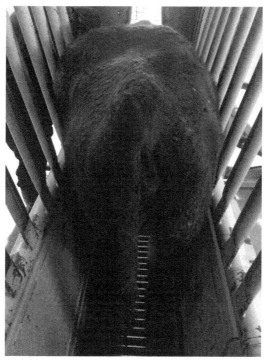

Fig. 1. Dorsal distention of the left flank of a cow consistent with a type 1 vagal indigestion.

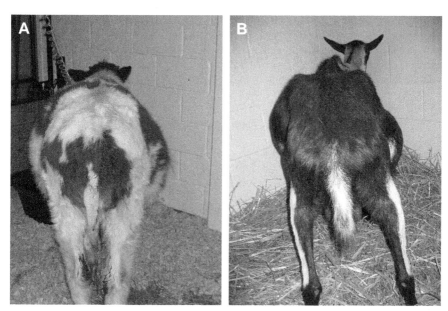

Fig. 2. Asymmetric, bilateral distension of a steer (*A*) and goat (*B*) consistent with type 2 or 3 vagal indigestion.

distension. In either case, the distension on the left is more diffuse and located in the middle to dorsal region of the flank ("apple" shaped), whereas the distension on the right is in the ventral flank ("pear" shaped). This combination leads to the description of these cows as "papple" shaped due to their asymmetric bilateral distension.

Bilateral ventral distension is generally due to fluid accumulation in the abdomen or uterus, and therefore, rarely gastrointestinal in origin (**Fig. 3**). Differentials for these animals include pathologic accumulations of fluid in the uterus due to placental or fetal abnormalities, peritoneal effusion, or uroabdomen. Appropriate history, rectal palpation, and abdominocentesis can be used to differentiate these, but this is beyond the scope of this article.

Abnormalities of rumen motility

Hypermotility of the rumen is a relatively uncommon finding, although in actuality it likely occurs quite frequently. In cases of early rumen distension, hypermotility may be noted as the moderate stretch receptors in the rumen wall are stimulated. The rumen continually senses this distension as a recent meal, and increases the rate of primary contractions in response to this distension. Therefore, in most cases of pathologic rumen distension, there is an early phase associated with rumen hypermotility.[13] Due to the early nature of the disease course and mild distension, it is unusual for an owner to present an animal for examination at this stage, and the hypermotility is missed. As the distension increases, the severe stretch then stops rumen contractions, and it is at this stage at which animals are typically examined.

Hypomotility is a much more common finding in clinically ill ruminants. As mentioned previously, systemic inflammation or increased sympathetic tone from a variety of causes will decrease rumen motility. Hence, most cases of rumen hypomotility are from causes outside the rumen. A thorough physical examination is necessary to rule out other causes of decreased rumen contractions. Hypomotility due to rumen diseases are most commonly associated with rumen distension or rumen acidosis. When the rumen is severely distended, rumen contraction rate will slow down and ultimately stop. Some disorders, traumatic reticuloperitonitis for example, may first disrupt normal motility, leading to rumen distension, which then further slows the contraction rate. Other disorders, such a physical obstruction of the omasal canal, lead to a primary rumen distension, and the distension ultimately slows and stops rumen contractions. This distinction is important prognostically, as cases with primary

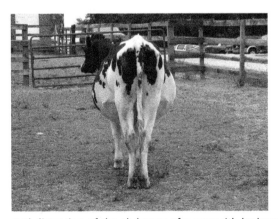

Fig. 3. Bilateral ventral distension of the abdomen of a cow with hydrops.

motility disorders are less likely to return to productivity after relieving the distension and underlying problem, whereas those with hypomotility due to distension are more likely to return to normal function after relieving the distension.

Disorders associated with rumen distension and dysmotility

Ruminants with both rumen distension and dysmotility typically are diagnosed with vagal indigestion, although rumen acidosis and rumen impactions also should be considered depending on the animal's abdominal shape, rumen fill, and dietary history. In spite of the name, clinical cases of vagal indigestion have been repeatedly shown to not involve the vagus nerve in most cases. Further, Hoflund's original description[14] of the disease based on experimental transection of the vagus nerve does little to guide diagnostic and therapeutic decisions. The classification scheme of 4 types of vagal indigestion by Ferrante and Whitlock[15] provide a more clinically useful approach to understanding these diseases and will be used here. No matter the underlying cause, the disease typically progresses from mild rumen distension leading to hypermotility, then progressive distension causes rumen hypomotility. At this point, the animal usually presents with severe rumen distension, decreased rumen contraction rate, and anorexia.

Type 1 vagal indigestion is associated with a failure of eructation. These animals present with gas distension of the dorsal left flank, and rumen hypomotility. This can occur due to a failure of secondary contractions, an inability to clear the cardia of fluid, failure of the cardia to open, or esophageal obstruction. A loss of secondary contractions appears to be relatively rare, although this may play a role in the bloat that can be seen in some calves with chronic respiratory disease. It is hypothesized that the vagus nerve can become inflamed in the thorax secondary to the respiratory disease. Bloat that is seen within laterally recumbent ruminants is due to fluid flooding the cardia, in spite of normal rumen motility. Similarly, the froth that can be created from consumption of legumes is sensed as fluid at the cardia, and prevents eructation. Damage to the rumen epithelium in the area of the cardia from rumenitis can damage the receptors responsible for sensing the presence of gas at the cardia, allowing it to open for eructation. Obstruction of the esophagus can occur from an intraluminal obstruction (swallowing an apple), an extraluminal mass (tracheobronchial lymphadenopathy in cases of respiratory disease), or a mass at the cardia (papilloma). Note that in all of these cases, the distension arises from a failure to eructate, not from an increased rate of gas production. Even with significant gas production from fermentation, the normal ruminant can increase eructation adequately to eliminate the gas.

Animals with type 2 vagal indigestion present with bilateral distension of the abdomen due to fluid accumulation in the rumen. The abdomen is distended at the midflank and dorsally on the left and ventrally on the right. On rectal examination, the classic finding of an "L"-shaped rumen is felt due to the significant expansion of the ventral sac toward the right flank. The fluid accumulation arises from a failure of rumen outflow with continued food and water intake and saliva production. The obstruction of the omasal orifice can be either functional or mechanical. Functional failures are most commonly due to traumatic reticuloperitonitis leading to inflammation and adhesions around the reticulum. Without normal reticular contractions, primary contractions are disrupted, and fluid is not aspirated into the omasal canal.[16] Other causes of peritonitis in the cranial abdomen including liver abscesses may present similarly.[17] Mechanical obstructions can occur secondary to consumption of a foreign body, including rope, hay netting, or placenta.[18] Masses including fibropapillomas and other neoplasias can also obstruct outflow.[19] In these cases, primary contractions are not disrupted initially, and they serve to maintain the foreign body lodged in the omasal orifice. Once the rumen becomes overly distended, then the rumen contractions stop.

Type 3 vagal indigestion presents similarly to type 2 in that the animal has the classic "papple" shape and fluid distension of the rumen. The difference is that the distension is due to a failure of abomasal motility and outflow. Reflux of abomasal fluid leads to the rumen distension, and the abomasum and rumen both contribute to the abdominal distension that is seen externally. The combination of abomasal and rumen distension leads to rumen hypomotility. Like type 2 vagal indigestion, type 3 also can be due to a functional or mechanical failure of abomasal motility. Functional causes include abomasal lymphosarcoma,[20] traumatic reticuloperitonitis,[16] and abomasal damage after an abomasal volvulus.[21] Roughly 15% of cattle with an abomasal volvulus will go on to develop abomasal motility disorders. This appears to be due to ischemic damage to the abomasal wall, peritonitis, and/or damage to the vagus nerve.[21] Mechanical obstructions here are less common, although lymphosarcoma and feed or sand impactions can also physically disrupt pyloric outflow. Iatrogenic causes should be considered, including inappropriately placed pyloropexy or incorrect placement of a toggle suture.

Type 4 vagal indigestion is a less well defined syndrome of partial pyloric obstruction or generalized ileus. These animals have less abdominal distension compared with those with type 2 or 3 vagal indigestion. A common reason for this presentation is late-term pregnancy, as the fetus may physically impede pyloric outflow or proximal intestinal motility.[22] Other causes are related to severe systemic disease, including hypocalcemia, peritonitis, septicemia, and enteritis leading to reduced intestinal motility.

Rumen acidosis is more thoroughly discussed in Nathan F. Meyer and Tony C. Bryant's article, "Diagnosis and Management of Rumen Acidosis and Bloat in Feedlots," in this issue, but is worth mentioning here as another cause of rumen distension and hypomotility. Due to the rapid production of volatile fatty acids from grain fermentation that exceeds the absorptive capacity of the rumen, water is pulled by osmosis into the rumen. This accumulation of fluid in the rumen causes a left-sided abdominal distension that may initially appear similar to a type 2 or 3 vagal indigestion. The abnormally low pH of the rumen fluid stops rumen contractions as the rumen attempts to slow fermentation. These animals with rumen acidosis will typically be more depressed and dehydrated than those with vagal indigestion, and examination of the rumen pH allows for easy differentiation of these diseases.

Animals with a rumen impaction will present with a firm, left-sided abdominal distension due to feed accumulation in the rumen. Rumen contraction rate will be variable depending on the degree of distension, and could range from increased to absent. The underlying pathogenesis of this disease could be either a lack of appropriate rumen microbial populations or feeding a low-quality, largely indigestible forage. The former can be seen in young animals who begin consuming large amounts of forage before developing a functional rumen or in an adult animal who has lost the normal rumen bacterial population after acidosis, anorexia, or antimicrobial administration. When fed indigestible forage, the rumen bacteria cannot adequately break down the plant material or the fermentation is excessively slow. This leads to an accumulation of fiber within the rumen as the animal continues to consume a large volume of feed material, yet cannot meet its nutritional needs. Hence, in chronic cases, animals will present with severe rumen distension but extremely poor body condition. The severe weight loss may be overlooked by owners due to the animal's large abdomen.[3]

Diagnostic Approach to Animals with Rumen Distension and Dysmotility

History and physical examination

When examining an animal with rumen distension and dysmotility, a complete physical examination will generally provide practitioners with a reasonably short list of differentials that can be further assessed with minimal diagnostic testing. Before examining the animal, it is useful to gather an appropriate nutritional and housing history. How much grain is fed? What is the quality of forage that is provided? Any exposure to legumes? Recent construction or building of fences? Evidence of trash or other potential foreign bodies in the pasture or animal's enclosure? Has the animal had a recent abomasal volvulus, pyloropexy, or toggle procedure? Then the animal is observed before restraint to properly assess abdominal contour, as described previously.

Rumen contraction rate and strength should be assessed by auscultation of the left paralumbar fossa. Most of these animals will have few or no rumen contractions. If the animal does have some contractions, simultaneous auscultation of the reticulum with palpation of the rumen will determine if the contractions are primary or secondary contractions. During the examination, particular attention should be paid to those potential diseases that can lead to vagal indigestion. A withers pinch should be performed. A lack of response could be due to any cause of cranial abdominal pain, although traumatic reticuloperitonitis is the classic disease associated with this finding. Other considerations include a ruptured liver abscess or a perforating abomasal ulcer. Practitioners may get some indication of the underlying problem if the cow responds more severely to sternal pressure on the right or left, as traumatic reticuloperitonitis will typically cause more pain on the left, whereas other causes are more likely located on the right. On auscultation of the thorax, is there evidence of respiratory disease or muffling of the heart associated with traumatic reticulopericarditis? Is there any lymphadenopathy that might be suggestive of lymphosarcoma? On rectal examination, the rumen size and texture is assessed to determine if there is fluid distension of the ventral sac. Also, the pregnancy status of the animal is determined, internal lymph nodes are palpated, and the viscera are palpated for evidence of peritonitis and adhesions.

ANCILLARY DIAGNOSTIC TESTING
Rumen Fluid Analysis

After completing the physical examination, passing a stomach tube is valuable diagnostically and therapeutically. In many cases of type 1 vagal indigestion, gas will be released when the tube is passed. With type 2 or 3 vagal indigestion, fluid may spontaneously reflux from the tube. If not, fluid should be siphoned off the rumen to reduce the distension and provide a sample for diagnostic evaluation. On collection of the fluid, the pH should be evaluated to rule out rumen acidosis. In cases of vagal indigestion, the pH will be normal (5.5–7.0) or slightly alkaline due to anorexia. The reflux of abomasal fluid with type 3 vagal indigestion is not sufficient to reduce rumen pH out of the normal range. When collecting rumen fluid orally, it is critical to collect several hundred milliliters of fluid to minimize the impact of saliva contamination on the pH. Excessive saliva contamination in a small volume sample will artificially elevate the pH due to the buffering capacity of ruminant saliva. A drop of the fluid should be placed on a microscope slide and evaluated at low magnification to assess protozoal activity. There should be numerous protozoa of varying sizes rapidly moving across the field. This can be used as a proxy measure of general microbial activity, as the protozoa appear to be more susceptible to changes in the rumen environment. In particular, the larger Holotrich protozoa appear to be especially sensitive to changes in the rumen environment.[23] Acidosis or prolonged anorexia in vagal indigestion are the most common causes of decreased protozoal numbers. This assessment needs to be done relatively rapidly, as these protozoa can be quite susceptible to changes in temperature and exposure to oxygen. Bacterial populations can be further investigated by Gram staining a sample of fluid, and measuring the methylene blue reduction time.

A sample of rumen fluid also should be strained for measurement of chloride content. In normal rumen fluid, the chloride content should be less than 30 mEq/L. Abomasal outflow obstructions (type 3 vagal indigestion) cause an increase in rumen chloride as the chloride secreted into the abomasum refluxes back into the rumen.[24] It remains sequestered there due to the rumen epithelium's relatively poor ability to absorb electrolytes. This finding is quite useful in differentiating type 2 and type 3 vagal indigestion, as they often present similarly. It has been demonstrated that acetate in the rumen fluid can falsely elevate chloride measurement when assessed using routine potentiometric blood chemistry analysis.[25] This interference is of less concern in animals with anorexia, as the acetate levels will be lower. Further, a chloride level less than 30 mEq/L can be reliably interpreted as normal, whereas an elevated rumen chloride concentration could be due to abomasal reflux or increased acetate levels. Therefore, it is critical to interpret rumen chloride concentrations in concert with blood chemistry analysis (**Table 2**).

Blood Chemistry Analysis

Assessment of serum chloride and bicarbonate can be useful in distinguishing between type 2 and 3 vagal indigestion for similar reasons as rumen chloride. Reflux of the chloride and subsequent sequestration in the rumen leads to a severe hypochloremia as the chloride is normally reabsorbed in the duodenum. Similarly, the hydrogen ions secreted into the abomasum to acidify the contents are associated with bicarbonate moving into the bloodstream. Normally, the bicarbonate from the bloodstream is then taken by the duodenum to neutralize the abomasal pH when ingesta enters the proximal small intestine. When this flow is disrupted, a severe metabolic alkalosis occurs as the bicarbonate remains in the circulation. Hence, animals with a type 3 vagal indigestion will have a severe hypochloremic metabolic alkalosis. Those with other rumen motility disorders may have similar electrolyte and acid-base derangements, but not to the same degree. The hypochloremic, metabolic alkalosis in these cases is associated with reduced abomasal motility due to anorexia and systemic disease. Other findings on the blood chemistry analysis also can be instructive, as an increase in globulins would suggest a chronic inflammatory process, such as traumatic reticuloperitonitis.

Ultrasound of the Reticulum

To definitively identify reticular contractions, it is helpful to use ultrasound to visualize the reticulum as auscultation can be difficult, and does not let one evaluate the strength of the reticular contraction.[26] The reticulum can be identified to the left of

Table 2 Rumen fluid analysis	
Color	Yellow-green to olive green depending on diet
pH	5.5–7
Protozoal activity	Abundant protozoa of different sizes
Methylene blue reduction	<5 min
Chloride	<30 mEq/L

midline, just caudal to the xiphoid. It will appear as a U-shaped structure, and only the wall can be seen due to the gas mixed into the ingesta. The cranial sac of the rumen will appear just caudal to the reticulum. The reticulum will have a biphasic contraction in which the first contraction is smaller, and the second completely collapses the reticular lumen as it moves dorsally. Identification of normal reticular contractions in cases of rumen distension suggests that the problem is less likely a functional motility disorder of the forestomach. A lack of reticular contractions, on the other hand, may suggest either a primary motility disorder or hypomotility due to rumen distension. Interestingly, many animals with rumen hypomotility will have reticular hypermotility, and this was particularly pronounced in cases of type 2 vagal indigestion.[27] Further, imaging of this area can identify abscesses, adhesions, or fluid accumulation associated with traumatic reticuloperitonitis.

Rumenotomy/Abdominal Exploratory

Abdominal surgery may ultimately be necessary to accurately diagnose the underlying disease in animals with rumen distension and dysmotility. This has the advantage of being both diagnostic and therapeutic. Before surgery though, one must determine if the animal most likely has a type 1 or 2 vagal indigestion versus a type 3 or 4. This distinction is important, as surgical diagnosis and correction of type 1 and 2 vagal indigestion is best accomplished through a left flank celiotomy and rumenotomy, whereas type 3 and 4 problems are best addressed from a right flank celiotomy and exploratory (**Table 3**).

TREATMENT OPTIONS

Treatment of the most these disorders associated with rumen distension and dysmotility are more thoroughly addressed in Robert J. Callan and Tanya J. Applegate's article, "Temporary Rumenostomy for the Treatment of Forestomach Diseases and Enteral Nutrition," Nathan F. Meyer and Tony C. Bryant's "Diagnosis and Management of Rumen Acidosis and Bloat in Feedlots" and Matt D. Miesner and Emily J. Reppert's "Diagnosis and Treatment of Hardware Disease," in this issue, and will commonly require a rumenotomy or abdominal exploratory as discussed previously. A few principles of therapy applicable to any of the previously discussed disorders are discussed as follows.

Table 3
Types of vagal indigestion

Type of Vagal Indigestion	Location of Abdominal Distension	Rumen Contents	Rumen Chloride	Serum Chloride	Serum Bicarbonate
Type 1: Failure of eructation	Dorsal left	Gas	Normal	Normal to mildly decreased	Normal to mildly increased
Type 2: Failure of rumen outflow	Dorsal left, ventral right	Fluid	Normal	Normal to mildly decreased	Normal to mildly increased
Type 3: Failure of abomasal outflow	Dorsal left, ventral right	Fluid	Increased	Moderate to severely decreased	Moderate to severely increased
Type 4: Partial failure of pyloric outflow/ proximal intestinal obstruction	Dorsal left, ventral right	Fluid	Normal to increased	Mild to moderately decreased	Mild to moderately increased

Emergency Treatment

Emergency treatment of severe rumen distension may be necessary even before complete evaluation. As the rumen becomes distended, the animal's ability to breathe is reduced as the rumen impedes normal movement of the diaphragm. Passage of a large-diameter orogastric tube should always be one's initial consideration, as this will allow passage of accumulated gas or fluid without the risk of peritonitis associated with rumen trocarization. A surfactant, such as poloxalene, can be administered at this time if there is any suspicion of a frothy bloat. Trocarization of the rumen can be performed in cases of extreme respiratory distress or if passage of an orogastric tube is not possible. A self-retaining, screw-in trocar is best, but no matter what type is used, owners should be made aware of the significant risk of peritonitis.

Transfaunation

For any of these diseases, there is likely to be an associated disruption of the rumen microbial populations. This disruption could be due to pH changes following rumen acidosis or due to prolonged anorexia in cases of vagal indigestion. Correction of the underlying cause of the motility disorder is key, but transfaunation with normal rumen fluid can speed the animal's return to normal productivity by replenishing the microbial populations. Drenching an adult bovine via an ororuminal tube (or adding directly to the rumen during a rumenotomy) with 10 to 16 L fresh rumen fluid appears to be clinically effective. Similarly, transfaunation of 1 to 4 L fresh rumen fluid in sheep and goats can reestablish normal microbial populations.[28]

SUMMARY

Rumen distension and dysmotility (most commonly hypomotility) are often found together in clinical cases. A thorough physical examination to determine the location of the rumen distension, assess the rumen contents, and careful auscultation of rumen contraction patterns will commonly provide the examiner with a relatively short differential diagnosis list. From here, rumen fluid analysis, ultrasound of the reticulum, and blood chemistry analysis can further guide surgical planning. Based on these findings, the practitioner can then make an informed decision concerning the surgical approach: left flank rumenotomy for rumen acidosis, type 1, or type 2 vagal indigestion or a right flank exploratory for type 3 or 4 vagal indigestion.

REFERENCES

1. Constable PD, Hoffsis GF, Rings DM. The reticulorumen: normal and abnormal motor function. Part I. Primary contraction cycle. Comp Cont Educ Pract Vet 1990;12:1008–14.
2. Constable PD, Hinchcliff KW, Done SH, et al. Clinical examination and making a diagnosis. In: Veterinary medicine. 11th edition. St Louis (MO): Elsevier; 2017. p. 1–28.
3. Garry F, McConnell C. Indigestion in ruminants. In: Smith B, editor. Large animal internal medicine. 5th edition. St Louis (MO): Elsevier; 2014. p. 777–88.
4. Membrive CMB. Anatomy and physiology of the rumen. In: Millen DD, Arrigoni MB, Pacheco RDL, editors. Rumenology. Basel (Switzerland): Springer; 2016. p. 1–38.
5. Herdt TH, Sayegh AI. Digestion: the fermentative processes. In: Klein B, editor. Cunningham's textbook of veterinary physiology. 5th edition. St Louis (MO): Elsevier; 2012. p. 331–59.

6. Braun U, Schweizer A. Ultrasonographic assessment of reticuloruminal motility in 45 cows. Schweiz Arch Tierheilkd 2015;157(2):87–95.

7. Waghorn GC. Relationships between intraruminal pressure, distension, and the volume of gas used to simulate bloat in cows. New Zeal J Agric Res 1991;34: 213–20.

8. Constable PD, Hoffsis GF, Rings DM. The reticulorumen: normal and abnormal motor function. Part II. Secondary contraction cycles, rumination, and esophageal groove closure. Comp Cont Educ Pract Vet 1990;12:1169–74.

9. Sellers AF, Stevens CE. Motor functions of the ruminant forestomach. Physiol Rev 1966;46:634–61.

10. Ruckebusch Y, Tomov T. The sequential contractions of the rumen associated with eructation in sheep. J Physiol 1973;235(2):447–58.

11. Dougherty RW, Habel RE, Bond HE. Esophageal innervation and the eructation reflex in sheep. Am J Vet Res 1958;19(70):115–28.

12. Clarke RT, Reid CS. Foamy bloat of cattle. A review. J Dairy Sci 1974;57(7): 753–85.

13. Constable PD, Hinchcliff KW, Done SH, et al. Diseases of the alimentary tract–ruminant. In: Veterinary medicine. 11th edition. St Louis (MO): Elsevier; 2017. p. 436–621.

14. Hoflund S. Untersuchungen über Störungen in den Funktionen der Wiederkäuermagen, durch Schädigungen des Nervus vagus verursacht. Svensk Veterinärtidskrift 1940;45(Suppl 1):1–59.

15. Ferrante PL, Whitlock RH. Chronic vagal indigestion in cattle. Comp Cont Ed 1981;3:S231–7.

16. Rehage J, Kaske M, Stockhofe-Zurwieden N, et al. Evaluation of the pathogenesis of vagus indigestion in cows with traumatic reticuloperitonitis. J Am Vet Med Assoc 1995;207(12):1607–11.

17. Doré E, Fecteau G, Hélie P, et al. Liver abscesses in Holstein dairy cattle: 18 cases (1992-2003). J Vet Intern Med 2007;21(4):853–6.

18. Braun U, Schweizer G, Flückiger M. Radiographic and ultrasonographic findings in three cows with reticulo-omasal obstruction due to a foreign body. Vet Rec 2002;150(18):580–1.

19. Gordon PJ. Surgical removal of a fibropapilloma from the reticulum causing apparent vagal indigestion. Vet Rec 1997;140(3):69–70.

20. Burton AJ, Nydam DV, Long ED, et al. Signalment and clinical complaints initiating hospital admission, methods of diagnosis, and pathological findings associated with bovine lymphosarcoma (112 cases). J Vet Intern Med 2010;24(4): 960–4.

21. Sattler N, Fecteau G, Hélie P, et al. Etiology, forms, and prognosis of gastrointestinal dysfunction resembling vagal indigestion occurring after surgical correction of right abomasal displacement. Can Vet J 2000;41(10):777–85.

22. Hussain SA, Uppal SK, Sood NK, et al. Clinico hemato biochemical findings, clinical management, and production performance of bovines with late pregnancy indigestion (type IV vagal indigestion). Vet Med Int 2014;2014:525607.

23. Ffoulkes D, Leng RA. Dynamics of protozoa in the rumen of cattle. Br J Nutr 1988; 59(3):429–36.

24. Kuiper R, Breukink HJ. Reticulo-omasal stenosis in the cow: differential diagnosis with respect to pyloric stenosis. Vet Rec 1986;119:169–71.

25. Cebra CK, Tornquist SJ, Vap LM, et al. A comparison of coulometric titration and potentiometric determination of chloride concentration in rumen fluid. Vet Clin Pathol 2001;30(4):211–3.

26. Braun U, Götz M. Ultrasonography of the reticulum in cows. Am J Vet Res 1994; 55:325–32.
27. Braun U, Rauch S, Hässig M. Ultrasonographic evaluation of reticular motility in 144 cattle with vagal indigestion. Vet Rec 2009;164(1):11–3.
28. DePeters EJ, George LW. Rumen transfaunation. Immunol Lett 2014;162(2 Pt A): 69–76.

Diagnosis and Treatment of Hardware Disease

Matt D. Miesner, DVM, MS*, Emily J. Reppert, DVM, MS

KEYWORDS

- Hardware • Rumen • Peritonitis • Pericarditis • Ruminant • Rumenotomy

KEY POINTS

- Cattle frequently ingest irregular objects with potential risk of rumeno-reticular damage and perforation, followed by peritonitis, pleuritis, and/or pericarditis, in addition to sepsis, restrictive adhesions, and/or abscess formation.
- Patients with hardware disease often present with client complaints of rumeno-reticular dysmotility (bloat), abdominal discomfort (colic), anorexia, lethargy, and weight loss (falling behind).
- During complete physical examination, heed evidence of pain localized to the cranioventral abdomen, abnormal auscultation findings consistent with rumen dysmotility, and pleural/peritoneal/pericardial effusion and inflammation.
- Ancillary diagnostics including an inflammatory leukogram, radiographs, and ultrasound are advantageous for diagnosis before exploratory laparotomy or rumenotomy.
- Treatment of hardware disease is directed at controlling infection and removing foreign bodies when possible: however, prevention should be the primary emphasis.

 Video content accompanies this article at http://www.vetfood.theclinics.com.

INTRODUCTION: NATURE OF THE PROBLEM

Traumatic reticuloperitonitis (TRP), resulting from penetration of the reticulum by a foreign body, is a common gastrointestinal (GI) disorder affecting adult dairy cattle and, less commonly, beef cattle. TRP results from the indiscriminate grazing habits and accidental ingestion of foreign bodies. Ingestion of a foreign body has 4 potential outcomes[1,2]:

1. Attachment to a previously administered magnet with no development of clinical disease
2. Penetration of the reticular wall without entering the peritoneal cavity, causing focal reticulitis and mild clinical disease

Disclosure Statement: The authors have nothing to disclose.
Veterinary Clinical Sciences, Kansas State University, 1800 Denison Avenue, Manhattan, KS 66506, USA
* Corresponding author. 103J Mosier Hall, Manhattan, KS 66506.
E-mail address: mmiesner@vet.k-state.edu

Vet Clin Food Anim 33 (2017) 513–523
http://dx.doi.org/10.1016/j.cvfa.2017.06.007

3. Perforation of the reticular wall and entrance to the peritoneal cavity causing acute localized TRP
4. Perforation of the reticular wall and entrance to the peritoneal or thoracic cavity resulting in pericarditis, myocarditis, abscessation, vagal indigestion, or other secondary disease

TRP remains a primary cause of vagal indigestion in cattle. Type II vagal indigestion (failure of omasal transport) is the most common type of vagal indigestion associated with TRP.

PATIENT HISTORY

In acute cases of TRP, animals typically develop clinical signs within 24 hours of the foreign body penetrating the reticular wall. Animals become anorexic, agalactic, reluctant to move, anxious, and in some cases may have an arched back.[2] Uncomplicated cases may resolve within 3 to 5 days after the initial acute episode. Resolution of disease is marked by increased appetite and return to normal milk production. In more complicated cases, development of clinical disease is protracted and clinical signs may remain static for days to weeks. Progression of disease may be the result of failure to localize the peritonitis or involvement of other organs resulting in ongoing disease. Cattle with chronic TRP may have decreased feed intake, milk production, and fecal output for prolonged periods of time.

PHYSICAL EXAMINATION

Early signs of TRP develop shortly after the foreign body perforates the reticular wall resulting in localized peritonitis. Acute disease caused by TRP is characterized by fever, anorexia, decreased to absent rumen contractions, and cranial abdominal pain. Evidence of cranial abdominal pain includes any of the following:

1. Absent ventroflexion with pressure applied to the withers
2. Grunt with pressure applied to the withers
3. Grunt with dorsal pressure applied to the xyphoid
4. Reluctance to move
5. Arched back when standing
6. Forelimbs held in an abducted position

TRP remains the most common cause of cranial abdominal pain in adult cattle. Differentials for cranial abdominal pain in cattle include[3]:

1. Localized peritonitis secondary to TRP, perforating abomasal ulcer, superficial hepatic abscess
2. Pleuritis
3. Pericarditis
4. Endocarditis

Other nonspecific clinical findings of TRP include abduction of the elbows, tachycardia, and tachypnea. Persistence or progression of clinical signs may indicate failure to contain the peritonitis or involvement of other structures. Sequela associated with TRP depends on the size, shape, and location of penetration. Penetration of the reticular wall and diaphragm can lead to bacterial seeding of the peritoneal, thoracic, and pericardial spaces resulting in peritonitis, pleuritis, and pericarditis. Inflammation, abscessation, and adhesions of the reticulum can lead to abnormal reticuloruminal motility and the development of vagal indigestion. Papple (L-shaped) abdominal contour is consistent with vagal indigestion. The spleen and the liver sit near the reticulum and can also be penetrated by a foreign body leading to splenitis and hepatitis. Local peritonitis that goes uncontrolled can lead to diffuse infection.

Ancillary Diagnostics

Diagnosing TRP in an animal in the acute stages of the disease that presents with acute onset of anorexia, decreased milk production, and reluctance to move is typically straight forward. The duration, severity, and involvement of other structures make definitively diagnosing chronic cases of TRP particularly challenging. A definitive diagnosis can be made by using ancillary diagnostics. Ancillary diagnostics used to support a diagnosis of TRP include complete blood count (CBC) with differential cell count and fibrinogen, haptoglobin, abdominocentesis, cranial abdominal radiography, and ultrasonography.

- CBC and fibrinogen
  - A white blood cell count (WBC) with neutrophilia seems to be most useful in acute cases of TRP. An elevated WBC characterized by neutrophilia and hyperfibrinogenemia are most consistently found in acute cases of TRP and are of limited utility in chronic cases of TRP.
- Total protein
  - Increased total protein has been evaluated as an indicator of TRP. Hyperproteinemia (due to increased globulin fraction) in an animal that is not dehydrated can be the response to subacute to chronic inflammation. Elevations in total protein may be used to confirm the likelihood of TRP. In a retrospective analysis of the sensitivity and specificity of total protein as a predictive value of TRP, animals with GI disease that have hypoproteinemia are unlikely to have TRP.[4] The same study also noted that 83.3% of cattle with elevated total protein concentration greater than 10.5 g/dL had TRP. However, few cattle with confirmed TRP had a hyperproteinemia that exceeded 10.5 g/dL. Hyperproteinemia is suggestive of TRP; however, the absence of hyperproteinemia does not rule out TRP.
- Fibrinogen and haptoglobin
  - A more recent study evaluating acute-phase biomarkers of inflammation associated with TRP measured fibrinogen and haptoglobin.[5] Fibrinogen concentrations were significantly higher in cattle with TRP compared with healthy control cows. There was no correlation between fibrinogen and WBC in cattle with TRP suggesting fibrinogen is a preferred marker for acute TRP. In animals with TRP, haptoglobin concentrations were significantly elevated when compared with controls and there was a positive correlation between haptoglobin and WBC. The investigators recommend interpreting haptoglobin and WBC simultaneously in animals suspected of having TRP.
  - Haptoglobin is not commonly measured and not readily available to most practitioners. Two studies have tried to determine the sensitivity and specificity of plasma fibrinogen needed to differentiate TRP from other GI disorders.[6,7] In one study, a plasma fibrinogen level of 570 mg/dL in animals showing signs consistent with TRP had a sensitivity of 32.1% and a specificity of 100%.[6] In a second study, researchers established cutoff values for plasma total protein and plasma fibrinogen when measured together. Cutoff points of 7.22 g/dL and 622.0 mg/dL for total plasma protein and plasma fibrinogen had a sensitivity of 88% and specificity of 86%.[7] In both studies, the sensitivity and specificity were variable and difficult to interpret. The clinical utility of fibrinogen to

differentiate an animal with TRP from an animal with other inflammatory conditions needs to be investigated further.

- Abdominocentesis
  - Peritoneal fluid analysis can be helpful in chronic cases whereby the leukogram and fibrinogen are inconclusive. The landmarks and technique for peritoneal fluid analysis have been previously described.[8] Characteristics of peritoneal fluid consistent with peritonitis include
    - Total nucleated cell count is greater than 6000 cells per microliter.
    - Total protein is greater than 3 g/dL.
    - Differential cell count reveals neutrophils greater than 40% and eosinophils less than 10%.
    - Failure to obtain fluid does not rule out peritonitis. The fibrinous response of cattle can rapidly wall off infection.
    - In cases of suspected pleuritis or pericarditis, thoracocentesis or pericardiocentesis can be performed.
- Radiographs
  - Cranial abdominal radiography is a useful imaging modality to diagnose of TRP. There have been several techniques described for obtaining a reticular image, including standing and recumbent methods.[9] Radiography is typically limited to referral practices with radiographic equipment powerful enough to obtain clear images of the bovine cranial abdomen. Radiographs are useful for identifying a metallic foreign body, the position of which may suggest penetration of the reticular wall.[10] Radiographs have also been used to determine the success or failure of magnet administration.[11] A study by Fubini and colleagues[10] evaluated the accuracy of radiographs compared with surgical findings in cows with TRP. The study found that radiographs are most accurate at identifying a foreign body and determining if the reticular wall has been penetrated. The investigators were unable to determine the utility of radiographs for identifying peri-reticular/hepatic abscessation secondary to TRP.
- Ultrasound
  - Reticular ultrasonography is useful for detecting abnormal motility associated with perireticular adhesions, perireticular abscessation, and peritoneal, thoracic, and pericardial effusion. Technique and interpretation of reticular ultrasonography have been recently reviewed.[12] Ultrasonographic findings suggestive of TRP include areas of mixed echogenicity and fibrin deposits between the reticulum and abdominal wall.[13] The size, shape, and location of a penetrating foreign body can also be imaged during ultrasound examination of the cranial abdomen.[13]

TREATING HARDWARE DISEASE

The clinician should consider options for removing the foreign body or, at minimum, preventing further trauma or penetration of the reticulum. The latter can be accomplished by administering a magnet orally that is then swallowed and attaches to metal foreign bodies still within the reticulum preventing further penetration. Often before surgical intervention, such as rumenotomy or thoracotomy, medical treatment should include basic supportive care through instituting proper antimicrobial measures, counteracting inflammation, replenishing fluid and electrolytes, and reducing pain. Prolong antimicrobial administration and monitor for secondary complications, such as ileus due to adhesions and vagal indigestion.

SUPPORTIVE CARE
Pharmacologic Treatment Options

Acute clinical cases involve a broad host of GI origin bacteria, leading to bacteremia and likely endotoxemia, whereas later chronic cases are more often *Trueperella pyogenes*. Tetracyclines and β-lactams are good choices against the broad spectrum of primarily anaerobes. Steroidal or nonsteroidal antiinflammatory drug (NSAID) therapy should be instituted early to treat against toxemia, inflammation, and pain and limit fibrin deposition and adhesion formation in later stages. Consider the hemodynamic changes associated with acute cases when administering potentially nephrotoxic medications, such as NSAIDs and tetracyclines, in hypovolemic states. Institute appropriate fluid therapy early. Consider multimodal pharmacologic approaches to pain management with the use of opiate drugs in addition to the antiinflammatories. When administering intravenous fluids, consider constant rate infusion of analgesic drugs.[14]

Nonpharmacologic Treatment Options

Magnets
The benefits of prophylactically placing a magnet in the reticulum to prevent TRP in cattle have been recognized since the 1950s whereby the practice could dramatically reduce the frequency of clinical signs. Occasionally, the length of the foreign body exceeded the length of early short magnets allowing trauma/perforation, so they were lengthened to 3 in to better protect the reticulum.[15] A magnet is a better preventive tool than therapeutic device but should still be a part of treating clinical disease. Assessment of magnet efficacy for reversing clinical disease is difficult without first definitively differentiating TRP from other conditions with similar clinical presentations. Because of imaging equipment limitations, diagnosis and recovery are most often based on clinical signs rather than objectively monitoring the foreign body path. It is possible that the foreign body fails to attach to the magnet, yet is walled off successfully with body defenses. One study showed that as long as the foreign body was free and on the ventral reticular floor, magnets attached 92% of the time, yet only 32% to 54% of the time when the foreign body showed evidence of penetration.[11] Various magnetic devices passed orally have been used to attempt retrieval of metallic foreign bodies followed by esophageal extraction.[16] Care should be taken to avoid esophageal trauma when using such devices.

Fluids
Acute, severe cases of hardware disease can lead to generalized septic peritonitis followed by hypovolemic shock. Inflammation and endotoxemia lead to hypoproteinemia due to increased vascular permeability with net loss of intravascular protein and influx into the peritoneal cavity. Cattle isolate the infection via omental patching and adhesion formation quickly and often present in later stages of disease. Plasma protein profiles often reflect this with hypoproteinemia due to negative acute-phase inflammatory proteins, such as albumin, early followed by hyperproteinemia with ensuing increase in positive acute-phase proteins (fibrinogen and globulins) later. Monitoring these parameters during treatment may assist in determining resolution or direct changes in course of treatment. To some extent, the location of foreign body penetration will affect the extent or dissemination of contamination before it can be walled off by the body, with penetrations into the supraomental recess being more severe. Fluid therapy is indicated and accomplished most effectively with large volumes of intravenous isotonic saline. A hypochloremic, hypokalemic, metabolic alkalosis is anticipated and due to ileus; oral fluids may be less effective. Additional fluid components, such as

potassium and magnesium, can be added in addition to plasma proteins through whole-blood or plasma transfusions.

Surgical Treatment Options

Rumenotomy

A left flank laparotomy and rumenotomy are performed to evaluate the extent of peritonitis and peri-reticular/rumen adhesions, attempt retrieval of intraluminal foreign bodies, and possibly lance peri-reticular abscesses into the lumen of the reticulum. In a recent retrospective study of cattle after rumenotomy for TRP, 26% were productive members of the herd, 40% had been sold based on production criteria, and 34% had either died or were euthanized 5 months to 5 years after surgery.[17] Causes of death or euthanasia were more commonly due to concurrent disease complications like preoperative peritonitis and vagal indigestion rather than rumenotomy in the population studied. In another study, 17 of 25 cattle with type II vagal indigestion due to peri-reticular abscessation survived and were productive following rumenotomy and intrareticular abscess drainage.[18] These findings highlight the reason prevention is key but also underscore early diagnosis and that rumenotomy, when carefully performed, can be accomplished successfully with relatively positive outcomes.

The most common complications of rumenotomy will be peritonitis, local soft tissue infection, subcutaneous emphysema, and dehiscence. These complications are minimized via adequate preoperative stabilization of patients, surgical field maintenance, approach, and technique. Preoperative antibiotics are encouraged and have been shown to limit postoperative infection.[19] Numerous options for rumenotomy technique have been presented in excellent detail elsewhere.[20–23] The authors prioritize considerations for rumenotomy based on evidence and experience to avoid complications and facilitate outcomes.

The surgeon should take into consideration individual arm length and patient size when locating the laparotomy incision in the left paralumbar fossa. The reticulum will need to be explored thoroughly with direct palpation of the mucosal lining, reticulo-omasal orifice, and evidence of adhesions. Position the incision low enough to reach the structures adequately. Roughly one hand width caudal to the last rib and 2 hands' width ventral to the transverse processes is the dorsal aspect of the approximately 20- to 25-cm skin incision. The surgeon will also decide on using a rumen board or suture technique for rumenotomy (**Fig. 1**). A rumen board speeds the process but may limit the arm reach to the reticulum in some situations. A major priority is to avoid abdominal contamination with rumen contents, so care should be taken to form a protected barrier through suture fixation technique or rumen board attachments. A protective shroud or drape is also recommended with either technique (**Fig. 2**). Comparison of suture and clamp techniques found that a complete rumen skin suture technique is superior to intermittent stay sutures for preventing contamination but will take the surgeon longer to perform.[23] Exploration of the reticulum will require accessible reach, time, repetitive entry into the stoma, and possibly removal of ruminal contents; therefore, a stable well-formed suture technique is preferred by the authors and is described.

The skin incision should be large enough to provide free passage of the surgeon's arm, recognizing that once the rumen is sutured to the skin, the stoma will be smaller than the laparotomy. The incision can be oriented from cranio-dorsal to caudo-ventral in parallel with the muscle fibers of the external abdominal oblique muscle to help positon the surgeon for easier access to the cranial rumen once the approach is made. Continue the incision into the abdomen taking care to identify the peritoneum and avoid inadvertent rumen puncture. Explore for evidence of rumeno-reticular adhesions

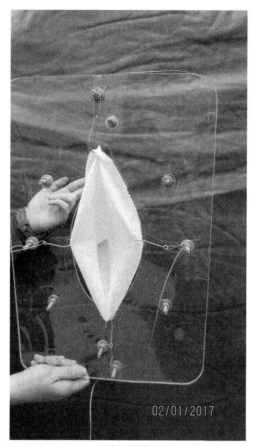

Fig. 1. Rumen board and attachment configuration.

with a sterile surgical sleeve, taking care not to disrupt and spread contamination via forceful breakdown of adhesions.

Remove the sterile sleeve and identify the portion of dorsal rumen sac to fix to the skin. Present sufficient rumen to the laparotomy site, and plan suture placement to provide a sufficient stoma for arm access maintaining several centimeters from the cut edge of the rumen to the sutured skin edge, as it will be necessary for closure. The pattern chosen to form the seal will be a combination of a Cushing pattern (regarding rumen wall suture placement) and a Connell-oriented skin placement. Suture bites of skin should be far enough from the skin edge to allow it to roll inward and invert, hiding the cut edge of skin. The suture type should be soft and nonabsorbable of at least size No. 3 that will not easily pull through the rumen wall; a cutting needle is recommended for easier penetration of the skin. The result will be a continuous seal inverting the epidermis to contact the serosal surface of the rumen (Video 1). At minimum, 2 continuous runs of this pattern should be performed, one on the cranial and one on the caudal side of the skin incision. The dorsal and ventral apex of the incision should receive special care to assure that a seal is formed, often sutured separately. The rumen is incised a few centimeters from the dorsal and ventral extent of the sutured seal. At this point a rumen shroud or drape can be

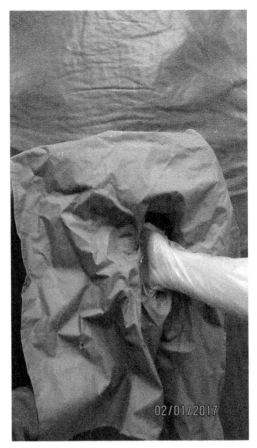

Fig. 2. Rumen shroud application.

positioned to add an extra layer of protection from contamination and prevent rumen trauma or suture disruption.

Explore the reticulum by following the dorsal rumen wall cranially to the reticulum identified by the honeycomb-shaped mucosa. Palpate and remove objects lying on the superficial mucosa, and brush the surface with the gloved hand feeling for fixed or protruding foreign bodies. Note the patients' response to focally painful areas. Grasp the rumeno-reticular pillar and begin to roll the reticular wall between the fingers, searching for buried foreign bodies deep in the wall of the reticulum as well as resistance in areas that may indicate adhesions. Note any areas of denuded or smooth mucosal surfaces or bulges possibly indicating peri-reticular abscesses. Identify the reticulo-omasal orifice, and take notice of the mucosa and reticular wall integrity of the ventral/medial reticulum as abscesses tend to form in this location. Abdominal ultrasonography has possibly already identified an abscess in this location; the goal is to now identify a location of soft, smooth, possibly bulging reticular mucosa for which to drain the abscess into the lumen. Suspect areas should be gently grasped, and attempt retraction to identify adhesions. Intraluminal ultrasound can be performed to confirm abscesses, or needle and syringe aspiration can help confirm abscesses. Once surgeons have identified an abscess and determined adequate adhesion to the reticulum to the best of their ability, the abscess can be lanced into the lumen of the reticulum. It is hoped that the abscess capsule contraction as well as return of reticular contractions will empty the abscess.

After exploration, remove the shroud and lavage the surgical site. Close the rumenotomy with absorbable suture material in a Cushing pattern. Release a portion of the proximal suture fixation, and begin a second Cushing layer to hide the rumen suture punctures from the fixation. Continue to release and suture until the rumenotomy is closed and released from the skin. Close the abdomen.

Thoracotomy
Septic pleuritis, pyothorax, or pericarditis can be approached through thoracotomy. A fifth or sixth partial rib resection can provide more thorough drainage of the area than trocar or catheter placement. Cost and recovery time should be considered with case management, and understand that localizing the foreign body for removal from the chest is rare. Unilateral septic pleuritis and pyothorax have a more favorable, yet guarded, prognosis than cattle with likely grave septic and restrictive pericarditis.[24] Unless the infection has compromised the normally complete mediastinum, cattle will be able to ventilate sufficiently with a hemithorax throughout the surgery and during second-intention healing of the wound. Therefore, the procedure can be performed standing under local anesthesia. General anesthesia can also be used. However, because of already existing reduction in cardiac output hemodynamic derangements, general anesthesia may carry a poorer chance of surgical survival than when done standing.[24] The authors prefer to postpone thoracotomy for several days if a rumenotomy has recently been performed looking for hardware or until patients prove to be stable with general supportive care.

The affected side is generously clipped and prepared for surgery. Tying the front limb forward will prevent interference during surgery. The fifth or sixth ribs are located by counting down from the last (13th) rib. Lidocaine is generously injected subcutaneously and intercostal, cranial and caudal to the targeted rib to be resected. A section of rib will be resected from the costochondral junction which is about the level of the elbow, and proximally about 10 cm or the width of the surgeon's hand. A linear skin incision is made directly over the rib to the periosteum. Incise the periosteum vertically and circumferentially proximal and distal to the section to be removed. The periosteum is then elevated along the incisions in circumferential fashion until an obstetric wire can be passed around the rib in both locations for removal. Some surgeons may only saw though the proximal rib and manually dislocate the rib from the costochondral junction distally.

After the rib section is removed, the pleura will need to be incised. Caution should be taken if the clinician suspects the pericardium is adhered to the pleura and consider slower decompression of the restrictive pericardial sac first to prevent shock from rapid decompression. Incise the pleura and lavage thoroughly. Place belt loop sutures of umbilical tape in several locations around the thoracotomy for application of a stent bandage to be changed often during postoperative recovery and wound management. Daily lavage is planned until wound closure, which could take weeks with second-intention healing. Consider partial closure or complete second-intention healing of the thoracotomy site. Partial or primary closure will limit healing time and drainage. Closure of the thoracotomy and a separate chest tube placement adjacent to the thoracotomy site with a unidirectional flow setup (Heimlich valve, Penrose tubing, or sterile surgical glove over the end) may also be used. The authors have noted that clinical tension pneumothorax can develop at the terminal stages of second-intention healing when the thoracotomy site is small and allows more dynamic pressure changes during respiration. During the last stages, a sterile plastic drape can be placed over the wound until granulation is complete.

SUMMARY

The indiscriminate eating habits of cattle can result in foreign body ingestion and the development of TRP. Diagnosis of acute disease can be straightforward, but chronic disease or development of sequelae can result in a diagnostic dilemma. Ancillary diagnostics, including blood work, radiographs, and ultrasound, can be used to aide in confirming the diagnosis. Some acute cases of TRP will respond to medical therapy alone, but more complicated cases may require surgical intervention including rumenotomy or thoracotomy.

SUPPLEMENTARY DATA

Supplementary data related to this article can be found online at http://dx.doi.org/10.1016/j.cvfa.2017.06.007.

REFERENCES

1. Ducharme NG. Surgery of the bovine forestomach compartments. Vet Clin North Am Food Anim Pract 1990;6(2):371–97.
2. Ward JL, Ducharme NG. Traumatic reticuloperitonitis in dairy cows. J Am Vet Med Assoc 1994;204:874–7.
3. Henninger RW, Mullowney PC. Anterior abdominal pain in cattle. Compend Contin Educ Vet 1984;6:S453–63.
4. Dubensky RA, White ME. The sensitivity, specificity and predictive value of total plasma protein in the diagnosis of traumatic reticuloperitonitis. Can J Comp Med 1983;47:241–4.
5. Kirbas A, Ozkanlar Y, Aktas MS, et al. Acute phase biomarkers for inflammatory response in dairy cows with traumatic reticuloperitonitis. Isr J Vet Med 2015;70:23–9.
6. Nazifi S, Ansari-Lari M, Asadi-Fardaqi J, et al. The use of receiver operating characteristic (ROC) analysis to assess the diagnostic value of serum amyloid A, haptoglobin and fibrinogen in traumatic reticuloperitonitis in cattle. Vet J 2009;182:315–9.
7. Jafarzadeh SR, Nowrouzian I, Khaki Z, et al. The sensitivities and specificities of total plasma protein and plasma fibrinogen for the diagnosis of traumatic reticuloperitonitis in cattle. Prev Vet Med 2004;65:1–7.
8. Fecteau G. Management of peritonitis in cattle. Vet Clin North Am Food Anim Pract 2005;21:155–71.
9. Ducharme NG, Dill SG, Rendano VT. Reticulography of the cow in dorsal recumbency: an aid in the diagnosis and treatment of traumatic reticuloperitonitis. J Am Vet Med Assoc 1983;182:585–8.
10. Fubini SL, Yeager AE, Mohammed HO, et al. Accuracy of radiography of the reticulum for predicting surgical findings in adult dairy cattle with traumatic reticuloperitonitis: 123 cases (1981-1987). J Am Vet Med Assoc 1990;197:1060–4.
11. Braun U, Gansohr B, Fluckiger M. Radiographic findings before and after oral administration of a magnet in cows with traumatic reticuloperitonitis. Am J Vet Res 2003;64:115–20.
12. Braun U. Ultrasonography of the gastrointestinal tract in cattle. Vet Clin North Am Food Anim Pract 2009;25:567–90. Table of Contents.

13. El-Esawy EE, Badawy AM, Ismail SF. Ultrasonographic diagnosis and clinical evaluation of the foreign body complications in the compound stomach of cattle and buffaloes. J Adv Vet Res 2015;5:109–20.
14. Abrahamsen E. Managing severe pain in ruminants. In: Anderson D, Rings D, editors. Current veterinary therapy food animal practice. 5th edition. St Louis (MO): Saunders/Elsevier; 2009. p. 570–4.
15. Carroll RE. The use of magnets in the control of traumatic gastritis of cattle. J Am Vet Med Assoc 1956;129:376–8.
16. Ozturk S, Aksoy O, Kilic E, et al. Removal of metallic foreign bodies using nasogastric magnetic tube in traumatic reticulitis in cows. Indian Vet J 2005;82: 1200–2.
17. Hartnack AK, Niehaus AJ, Rousseau M, et al. Indications for and factors relating to outcome after rumenotomy or rumenostomy in cattle: 95 cases (1999-2011). J Am Vet Med Assoc 2015;247:659–64.
18. Fubini SL, Ducharme NG, Erb HN, et al. Failure of omasal transport attributable to perireticular abscess formation in cattle: 29 cases (1980-1986). J Am Vet Med Assoc 1989;194:811–4.
19. Haven ML, Wichtel JJ, Bristol DG, et al. Effects of antibiotic prophylaxis on postoperative complications after rumenotomy in cattle. J Am Vet Med Assoc 1992; 200:1332–5.
20. Lozier JW, Niehaus AJ. Surgery of the forestomach. Vet Clin North Am Food Anim Pract 2016;32:617–28.
21. Niehaus AJ, Anderson DE. Ruminant surgery. Vet Clin North Am Food Anim Pract 2016;32:xiii–xiv.
22. Niehaus AJ. Rumenotomy. Vet Clin North Am Food Anim Pract 2008;24:341–7.
23. Dehghani SN, Ghadrdani AM. Bovine rumenotomy: comparison of four surgical techniques. Can Vet J 1995;36:693–7.
24. Ducharme NG, Fubini SL, Rebhun WC, et al. Thoracotomy in adult dairy cattle: 14 cases (1979-1991). J Am Vet Med Assoc 1992;200:86–90.

Temporary Rumenostomy for the Treatment of Forestomach Diseases and Enteral Nutrition

Robert J. Callan, DVM, MS, PhD*, Tanya J. Applegate, DVM

KEYWORDS

- Rumen • Forestomach • Rumenostomy • Fistula • Enteral feeding • Bloat
- Obstruction • Foreign body

KEY POINTS

- Temporary rumenostomy is a useful procedure for management of chronic rumen tympany, rumen distension, rumen dysbiosis, and enteral feeding or medication administration.
- Temporary rumenostomy has minimal postsurgical management and complications directly related to the surgery are uncommon.
- The rumenostomy stoma often closes by second intention in 3 to 4 weeks.
- Surgical closure of the rumenostomy can be performed if early closure is warranted or if the stoma does not close by second intention.

INTRODUCTION

The unique anatomic and functional characteristics of the forestomach in ruminants and the first gastric compartment in pseudoruminants (New World camelids) allow the surgical placement of a permanent or temporary portal or stoma into these compartments for medical treatment and research studies. The term ostomy refers to the surgical placement of a permanent or temporary opening between 2 hollow organs or between a hollow organ and the external body surface. Alternatively, the term otomy refers to the act of incising into a hollow organ.

A rumenostomy is a surgical procedure that results in an opening between the lumen of the rumen and the surface of the abdominal wall. The term rumen fistula is

Disclosure: The authors have nothing to disclose.
Livestock Medicine and Surgery, Department of Clinical Sciences, College of Veterinary Medicine and Biomedical Sciences, Colorado State University, 300 West Drake Road, Fort Collins, CO 80523-1678, USA
* Corresponding author.
E-mail address: Robert.Callan@colostate.edu

often mistakenly used instead of rumenostomy. Technically, a fistula is a communication that is not intentionally created. In pseudoruminants such as llamas and alpacas, the major fermentation organ is the first gastric compartment and the proper term is a first compartment gastrostomy.

Surgical rumenostomy (or gastrostomy) is a useful procedure that allows both the egress of rumen gas and contents and the delivery of rumen microflora (transfaunation), medications, and feed directly into the rumen.[1,2] A Permanent rumenostomy is generally fitted with a rubber cannula and provides long-term access to the rumen contents, particularly for collection of rumen fluid for transfaunation. Procedures for traditional rumenostomy and cannulation are well described.[1-3] The temporary rumenostomy is more common for medical treatment of patients with forestomach indigestion, tympany, or dysbiosis. They are also used for direct enteral feeding. When the rumenostomy is no longer needed, it can be allowed to close by second intention, or it can be surgically closed. This article discusses the indications, surgical procedure, enteral feeding, management, and closure of a temporary rumenostomy.

INDICATIONS

Temporary rumenostomy can be performed in any ruminant and is a useful surgical procedure in cattle, sheep, and goats. A similar procedure can also be performed in New World camelids (llamas and alpacas) but in these species the procedure is technically a temporary gastrostomy of the first gastric compartment. The decision to perform a temporary rumenostomy is based on multiple considerations of the underlying problem and the therapeutic goal. In one retrospective study, the underlying disease process in 24 cattle that underwent therapeutic temporary rumenostomy included vagal indigestion (3), pneumonia (5), abomasal impaction (2), pharyngitis or esophagitis (2), and lymphoma (1).[4] There are 4 general medical indications for which a rumenostomy may be considered: (1) to relieve rumen distension, (2) for removal or lavage of rumen contents, (3) to restore normal rumen microflora, and (4) for enteral feeding or repeated enteral medications. In many cases, multiple indications and therapeutic goals may be present for an individual patient.

Rumen distension and dysmotility are discussed in depth in Derek Foster's article, "Disorders of Rumen Distension and Dysmotility," in this issue and in other references.[2,5] Generalized rumen distension is evident by gross enlargement of the left abdomen, and in some cases also the right ventral abdomen. Rumen distension may be caused by abnormal forestomach motility, intestinal obstruction, generalized ileus, or abnormal contents (frothy bloat) and results in excessive accumulation of gas, ingesta, or fluid in the rumen (**Box 1**). A rumenostomy may be performed to relieve rumen distension as an adjunct to other treatments. In most cases a rumenostomy is not performed until after other medical or surgical treatments are attempted and are unsuccessful in relieving the rumen distension. It is important to understand that even if the underlying disease is corrected, normal forestomach motility may not return until rumen distension is resolved. Immediate relief of rumen distension benefits the patient by decreasing the abdominal pressure that impedes both respiratory and cardiovascular function. In cases in which the underlying medical condition is already resolved, relief of rumen distension and establishment of normal rumen microflora can result in improved forestomach motility and appetite.

Relief of rumen gas accumulation (gas bloat) should first be attempted by passage of a stomach tube. However, frequent repeated intubation may not be practical in cases of chronic recurrent gas bloat and rumen tympany. Recurrent ruminal tympany is observed in some calves with acute and chronic respiratory disease. The cause is

---

Box 1
Causes of generalized rumen distension and dysmotility

- Obstruction of the esophagus or cardia (foreign body or mass)
- Extraesophageal mass (thymoma, thymic lymphosarcoma, mediastinal lymph node)
- Esophageal myopathy (megaesophagus)
- Forestomach indigestion and dysbiosis
- Rumen acidosis
- Reticulo-omasal obstruction (foreign body, mass, omasal impaction, liver abscess)
- Traumatic reticuloperitonitis or reticular abscess
- Indigestible forage (hay belly)
- Ineffective primary or secondary rumen contractions
- Pyloric obstruction (right displaced abomasum, abomasal volvulus, pyloric lymphosarcoma, hairball, foreign body, abomasal impaction, late term pregnancy)
- Generalized intestinal ileus (peritonitis, hypocalcemia, enteritis)

---

not fully understood but is proposed to be secondary to enlargement of mediastinal lymph nodes that inhibit eructation, or dysfunction of the vagus nerve caused by intra-thoracic inflammation. Rumenostomy can provide short-term to long-term relief while the underlying cause of rumen dysfunction is treated and time is provided to resolve the conditions causing rumen tympany.

In cases of accumulated ingesta or fluid, a Kingman tube (large-bore stomach tube) may be used to decompress the rumen (**Fig. 1**). However, this is not always successful and a rumenostomy provides a means to effectively decompress the rumen while additional medical or surgical treatment is undertaken to resolve the underlying cause. Rumen distension with fluid or ingesta increases the risk of regurgitation and aspiration in animals undergoing recumbent procedures or general anesthesia. This risk of regurgitation can be reduced with decompression by rumenostomy. Decompression of the rumen before exploratory celiotomy also improves the ability to explore and manipulate abdominal organs during surgery.

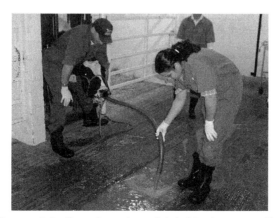

Fig. 1. Use of a Kingman tube (large-bore stomach tube) to decompress the rumen of a cow with vagal syndrome.

Reticulo-omasal foreign body obstruction is particularly difficult to diagnose in ruminants without access to the rumen contents. A full exploratory rumenotomy provides the best access to the rumen contents in cases of suspected foreign body. However, obstructing foreign bodies consisting of baling twine, plastic, and other materials are sometimes identified and removed when performing a temporary rumenostomy on calves and goats with nonspecific rumen distension. If a foreign body obstruction with these types of materials is suspected along with other causes for forestomach indigestion, then a rumenostomy may be a suitable diagnostic and treatment procedure that is less costly and time intensive than a full rumenotomy.

A temporary rumenostomy can be an alternative to a full rumenotomy when it is desired to remove the contents of the rumen (**Box 2**). This procedure may be indicated in situations of toxin ingestion, grain overload, or when the rumen contents do not support normal forestomach function. Removal of large amounts of feed material is more easily performed with a rumenotomy, particularly in adult cattle. Although a full rumenotomy gives better access to completely empty the rumen, this may not be a feasible procedure, particularly if multiple animals are affected. A rumenostomy can be performed more quickly and this is beneficial if the procedure needs to be performed for multiple animals with grain overload or ingestion of a toxin.

Following rumenostomy, the rumen can be partially emptied. This procedure is easier in calves and small ruminants than in adult cattle. Manual pressure on the ventral abdomen pushes the ingesta and fluid to the rumenostomy site where it can be physically removed or flushed out. A stomach tube or hose can also be used to lavage the rumen and, if needed, siphon contents that have settled to the bottom of the rumen. In cases of hay belly, removal of as much of the poor-quality forage as possible speeds resolution of the problem. Removal of this material often requires manually grasping the feed with forceps (ie, sponge forceps) and pulling it through the rumenostomy stoma.

Alteration in normal forestomach microflora (dysbiosis) can be either a cause or a result of abnormal forestomach motility and distension. Rumen fluid analysis is a simple and effective way to quickly evaluate general protozoal and bacterial health in the forestomach (See Dusty W. Nagy's article, "Diagnostic Approach to Forestomach Diseases," in this issue).[5,6] A rumen fluid analysis includes the evaluation of color, consistency, odor, pH, sedimentation time, reduction activity (methylene blue reduction test), and microscopic evaluation of protozoa and bacteria.

In cases of acute primary forestomach dysbiosis, rumen fluid transfaunation by stomach tube often restores functional forestomach microflora with a single treatment. However, repeated transfaunation may be required to restore normal microbial activity when the forestomach dysbiosis is chronic (rumen drinkers, rumen putrefaction) or is secondary to other forestomach or systemic disease. In these cases, rumenostomy can aid in treatment by providing a means to remove the abnormal rumen

---

Box 2
Indications for emptying rumen contents

- Rumen acidosis
- Ingested toxins (eg, toxic plants, lead)
- Rumen putrefaction
- Hay belly
- Foreign body

contents and also provide repeated rumen fluid transfaunation and nutritional support. A temporary rumenostomy provides an alternative to full rumenotomy for the removal of forestomach contents in cases of rumen acidosis, rumen putrefaction, and hay belly. Although a rumenotomy provides greater access and allows near-complete emptying of rumen contents, it is a much more involved surgical procedure. With a temporary rumenostomy, the rumen contents are allowed to be expelled over a longer period of time and repeated rumen fluid transfaunation can be easily performed (**Box 3**).

Supportive forced enteral feeding may be considered as adjunctive care in animals that have normal forestomach and distal intestinal function but the underlying disease condition is limiting feed intake. Enteral nutrition is challenging in ruminants because of the difficulty in administering forage and feeds of appropriate digestibility and fiber length through a stomach tube. The temporary rumenostomy is an effective procedure to allow enteral feeding because the size of the stoma can be selected to support the delivery of chopped forages and pelleted feeds directly into the rumen (**Box 4**).[7,8]

Permanent and temporary rumenostomy procedures are also used in ruminant research. The rumenostomy provides a continuous portal both to sample rumen contents and to deliver drugs and maintain monitoring devices within the rumen. Endoscopic evaluation of the forestomach of ruminants[9] and first gastric compartment of camelids can also be performed through a rumenostomy. Procedures for placing and maintaining abomasal sampling and monitoring devices with the aid of a rumenostomy are described.[10]

SURGICAL PROCEDURE

There are several descriptions of the temporary rumenostomy (rumen fistula) procedure, each with slight differences.[1,2,11] There is no indication from the literature that these differences significantly alter the outcome or adverse complications. Because this is a clean contaminated surgical procedure, preoperative antibiotics should be considered. Acceptable antibiotics include, but are not limited to, penicillin, ampicillin, ceftiofur, and oxytetracycline. Perioperative nonsteroidal antiinflammatory drugs such as flunixin meglumine or meloxicam should also be considered. In many cases, the patient is already receiving these treatments for the underlying condition.

The left paralumbar fossa is clipped and prepared for aseptic surgery. Sedation is rarely necessary and the animal can be restrained in a chute or standing with halter restraint (sheep, goats, calves, camelids). If possible, it is helpful to pass a stomach tube and relieve any gas distension of the rumen before surgery. This procedure can also be done with a needle before incising the abdominal wall. Either a

---

Box 3
Causes of forestomach dysbiosis

- Rumen acidosis (see Emily Snyder and Brent Credille's article "Diagnosis and Treatment of Clinical Rumen Acidosis," in this issue)
- Rumen putrefaction
- Rumen drinkers
- Forestomach motility disorders
- Secondary to other systemic disease
- Ingested toxins

Box 4
Indications for forced enteral feeding in ruminants and camelids

- Oral-facial trauma or fractures
- Esophageal trauma
- Megaesophagus
- Hepatic lipidosis
- Chronic central neurologic disease
- Tongue infections (ie, wooden tongue) or trauma
- Dysphagia caused by neuromuscular disease (ie, listeriosis, tetanus)
- Other systemic disease

---

paravertebral (proximal or distal) or inverted L block is suitable for local anesthesia.[12] Draping the site is helpful to minimize contamination of suture but is not required. An elliptical[1] or circular[2,11] (**Fig. 2**A) skin incision is made centrally in the dorsal third of the left paralumbar fossa. The size of the incision is based on the objectives of the procedure. If the procedure is being performed to relieve chronic rumen gas tympany, then the rumenostomy can be as small as 2 cm in diameter to simply produce a vent for excess gas. If the objective is to remove significant rumen contents, or to administer medications or enteral nutrition, then the incision should be large enough to accept an appropriately sized plastic, polyvinyl chloride (PVC), or rubber cannula. A syringe case (20–60 mL) can be used to make a convenient rumenostomy cannula (**Fig. 3**).

Following the skin incision, the subcutaneous tissue can be incised away with scissors. The body wall is opened in one of several fashions. The muscular layers of the abdominal wall and peritoneum can be punctured using straight hemostats.[11] The hole in the abdominal wall is then expanded by opening the jaws of the hemostat in different orientations until it is nearly as large as the skin incision. Alternatively, the abdominal muscle layers can be tented and incised vertically[1] or a circular portion of muscle can be removed using Mayo scissors (see **Fig. 2**B). Care must be taken not to cut into the rumen at this time, particularly if there is ruminal distension. A needle can be used to decompress the rumen if there is gas tympany. In addition, the peritoneum is incised (see **Fig. 2**C). At this time, the peritoneum and transverse abdominis muscle may be sutured to the deep dermis using absorbable suture.[1] This step is to provide an extra protection from rumen fluid contamination of the surrounding abdominal wall musculature and local cellulitis, and is optional based on surgeon preference.

Once the abdominal cavity is entered, the rumen wall should be apparent (see **Fig. 2**C). The rumen wall directly beneath the incision is grasped with hemostat forceps or a towel clamp, tented through the incision, and tacked in place with 3 to 4 equally spaced mattress stay sutures securing the rumen wall in contact with the skin (see **Fig. 2**D). The rumen wall is now sutured to the margins of the skin incision (see **Fig. 2**E). This step can be performed either before incising the rumen wall[1] or after incising the rumen.[2,11] The risk of local tissue contamination is increased if the rumen wall is incised before suturing to the skin but this method may allow better side-to-side apposition of the rumen wall margin with the skin. Multiple suture patterns have been described, including horizontal or vertical mattress,[2] a combination of Cushing in the rumen wall and simple continuous in the skin,[1] simple interrupted,[11] or a combination of these methods. Suture spacing should be very close in order to minimize leakage of rumen fluid into the subcutaneous tissues and abdominal musculature. Simple

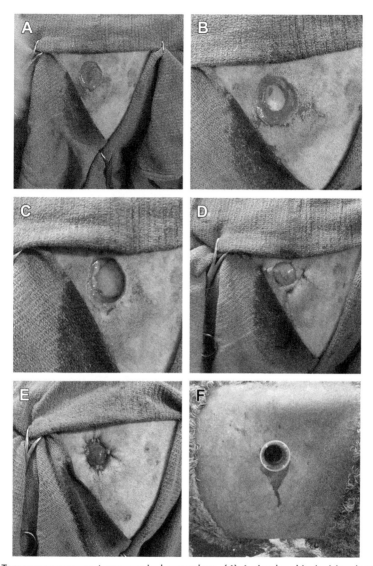

Fig. 2. Temporary rumenostomy surgical procedure. (*A*) A circular skin incision is made in the central dorsal one-third of the left paralumbar fossa. (*B*) The abdominal wall musculature is dissected to the peritoneum. (*C*) The peritoneum is incised and the rumen is observed within the abdomen. (*D*) The rumen wall is secured to the skin with 4 equidistant stay sutures. (*E*) The rumen wall is tightly sutured to the skin margins. (*F*) The rumen wall is incised and a syringe case cannula is secured with 2 stay sutures.

continuous patterns should be periodically tied around the circumference of the stoma so that the opening is not constricted with a purse string.

If the rumenostomy is going to be used for removal of contents or administration of medications or feed, it is preferable to secure a cannula in the stoma. A cannula can be easily made from a syringe case (see **Fig. 3**), PVC pipe, or commercial rubber cannula (Bar Diamond, Inc, www.bardiamond.com). When using a syringe case or PVC pipe,

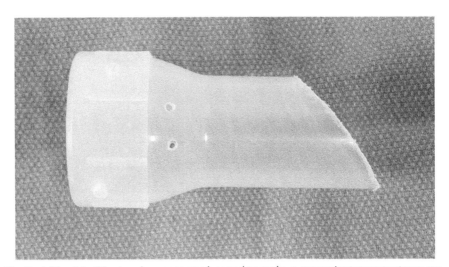

Fig. 3. A 20-mL to 60-mL syringe case can be used to make a convenient rumenostomy cannula. The syringe case is cut with a beveled end and the edges are filed smooth. From 2 to 4 pairs of holes are placed along the flange using a drill or a 14-g needle to accept stay sutures to hold the cannula in place. Two holes (4.8-mm diameter) are drilled through the cap and case with the cap in place. Zip-tie or paper-clip retainers can be placed through these holes to hold the cap in place when desired.

the cannula is secured with 2 to 4 stay sutures (see **Fig. 2**F). The cap of the syringe case can be used to decrease leakage of rumen contents (**Fig. 4**).

Following completion of the surgery, it may be indicated to evacuate as much of the rumen contents as possible, particularly in cases of rumen acidosis, rumen putrefaction, toxin ingestion, or severe rumen distension. This evacuation can be accomplished by applying manual pressure to the ventral abdomen. The rumen can also be lavaged with warm water and a stomach tube or hose. If rumen contents are removed, it is recommended to refill the rumen with a slurry of fresh rumen fluid and fiber from a donor animal (**Fig. 5**).

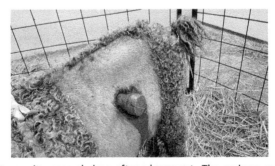

Fig. 4. Rumenostomy site several days after placement. The syringe case cap is used to decrease fluid leakage but some leakage occurs around the margins of the syringe case. Povidone iodine ointment or Vaseline can be used on the skin beneath the rumenostomy to decrease tissue irritation.

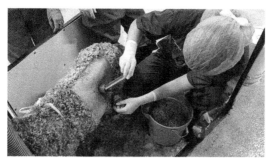

Fig. 5. Feeding of a rumen fluid and fiber slurry.

Reticulorumen foreign bodies may be identified while removing the rumen contents. If foreign body obstruction is a differential, attempts should be made to look for and remove these foreign objects. Sponge, Carmalt, or 90° forceps are useful instruments to grasp and remove these foreign materials (**Fig. 6**).

ENTERAL FEEDING

Methods for enteral feeding using a rumenostomy in cattle have been described.[7,8] The options for enteral feeding and fluid therapy vary based on the underlying medical condition, clinical status of the animal, and nutritional needs of the patient. In one study, successful enteral support was provided to 3 adult cows using a mixture of commercial dairy cow grain and alfalfa pellets targeting nutritional needs based on the National Research Council (NRC) nutrient requirements of daily net energy for each individual animal.[8] In addition, each animal in that study received individual fluid therapy, with water being a minimal need and specific electrolytes or minerals added

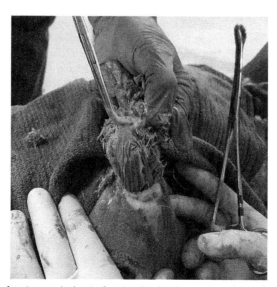

Fig. 6. Removal of twine and plastic foreign body obstruction through the rumenostomy stoma.

as indicated by blood work. In another report, enteral feeding was performed with chopped alfalfa hay and commercial concentrate.[7]

Enteral feeding may be accomplished via a combination of concentrates, pelleted feeds, ground forages, and slurries of rumen fluid and fiber. The feed combinations can be fed dry with added water, or as a gruel. The use of NRC-specific guidelines for maintenance energy requirements may help guide specific feeding regimens for a given feedstuff.[7,8] However, the ability to meet a maintenance energy requirement may be limited for certain production stages (eg, lactating dairy cows). The major challenge is delivering a sufficient volume of fluid through the rumenostomy without overloading the rumen. At least twice-daily feedings are necessary and, in most cases, more frequent feedings are required in order to provide adequate feed intake. A general rule is to attempt to provide 2% of body weight in dry matter intake of high-quality forage and concentrate per day.

The concentrate portion (including pelleted feeds) of the diet should not exceed 30% of the dry matter intake unless the animal is sufficiently adapted to the higher concentrate. Feeding large amounts of concentrates or pelleted feed increases the potential for digestive upset and rumen acidosis. Careful monitoring of gastrointestinal function and rumen pH is strongly advised when high-energy readily digestible feedstuffs such as concentrates, pelleted feeds, or finely ground forage are fed. In these types of diets, it is very easy for rumen acidosis to develop.

Rumen acidosis was found to be a significant complication when feeding a complete pelleted diet in a postoperative period in sheep.[13] In this study, sheep undergoing a surgical orthopedic procedure were fed either a complete pelleted diet or timothy grass hay. Rumen pH, rumen motility, and feed intake were monitored. The group receiving an exclusively pelleted diet postoperatively developed signs of ruminal acidosis, including reduced rumen motility, reduced rumen pH, reduced live rumen protozoa, and anorexia. Although this study was not directly evaluating a rumen cannula procedure, it shows that a complete pelleted diet had increased frequency of postoperative complications, with ruminal acidosis being a primary concern.

Administration of fresh rumen fluid is considered an effective method of transfaunation and is thought to be beneficial in the treatment of general rumen indigestion and rumen dysbiosis.[5,6] In one study, cows that received rumen fluid after surgical correction of left displaced abomasum had higher dry matter intake, higher milk production, and lower beta-hydroxybutyrate levels than those that did not.[14] In the sheep study described earlier, sheep that developed indigestion and subclinical rumen acidosis were effectively treated via rumen transfaunation.[13] Given the variety of conditions that may lead to the placement of a temporary rumenostomy, it is logical that inclusion of rumen fluid and rumen fiber in the feeding of patients with a rumenostomy is beneficial, and perhaps even essential, for the health of the rumen and patient. The rumen microflora is essential for healthy rumen function, but, additionally, other constituents, such as volatile fatty acids, bicarbonate buffers, proteins, and other unknown factors, may provide beneficial effects.

MANAGEMENT

The surgical site requires at least minimal daily care in the immediate postoperative period (10–14 days). Daily care should include assessment of the cannula, evaluation for postoperative complication (eg, inflammation, abscess formation, dehiscence), and cleaning of the surrounding skin. Topical antiseptic such as povidone iodine ointment can be applied to the surgical incision to protect it and decrease the risk of incisional infection. Povidone iodine ointment or Vaseline can also be placed on the skin below the rumenostomy site to minimize skin scalding.

Care should be taken to assess the patient daily for the potential development of rumen acidosis, particularly if grain or pelleted feed is included in the enteral ration. Lack of long-stem roughage and increased easily digestible carbohydrates predispose patients to development of rumen acidosis. Monitoring the rumen pH is indicated in these situations and should be performed on a daily basis when initially beginning enteral feeding of grain or pelleted diets. Once stable, periodic checks are prudent to continue for an extended period of time.

The most common complications associated with rumen surgery, including rumenotomy and rumenostomy, include incisional infection, seroma, dehiscence, and peritonitis.[2,4] A retrospective study describing outcome of rumenotomy or rumenostomy in cattle reported overall short-term complication rates of 15%.[4] The most common complications of temporary rumenostomy in the 30-day postoperative period were incisional problems (1 of 24; 4%) and death, euthanasia, or removal from the herd (2 of 24; 8%). Long-term (5 months to 5 years) outcomes for temporary rumenostomy were reported for 18 animals and included removal from the herd (4), and death or euthanasia (9). Removal from the herd was a result of poor performance caused by the primary disease process. Cause of death or reason for euthanasia was highly variable and often related to disease processes and not directly related to the rumenostomy.

CLOSURE

When the rumenostomy is no longer needed, it can be allowed to close by second intention or by surgical closure. If a cannula is present, it should be removed. If excessive leakage of rumen contents is a concern, the cannula can be replaced by successively smaller cannulae as the stoma slowly contracts. It generally takes 3 to 4 weeks for a rumenostomy to close by second intention.

In some instances, the stoma does not fully close by second intention and becomes a chronic rumen fistula. Also, some clients choose to speed the closure of the rumenostomy because of the continued rumen fluid drainage. In these cases, surgical closure is indicated. Simple closure can be attempted by freshening the margins of the stoma with a scalpel blade and then suturing the margins closed. A single-layer or purse-string closure generally fails. If this method is attempted, it is recommended to place both an internal and external layer of sutures to promote closure.

Full surgical resection of the rumenostomy site is recommended when other methods have failed or to ensure closure on the first try. The rumenostomy is dissected from the abdominal wall and the abdomen is entered, allowing complete resection of the site, and primary closure of the rumen wall, abdominal wall, and skin. To perform the surgery, clip and aseptically prepare the left paralumbar fossa. Analgesia may be provided with a paravertebral or inverted L block.

The rumenostomy is sutured closed to minimize rumen fluid leakage (**Fig. 7**A). Two stay sutures are placed above and below the stoma for traction. An elliptical skin incision is made around the rumenostomy stoma and continued through the abdominal musculature to the peritoneum (see **Fig. 7**B). Care must be taken to identify the layers that are being incised and prevent inadvertent entry into the rumen. Once the peritoneum is identified, it is incised with scissors and the abdominal cavity is entered. Two additional stay sutures are placed in the rumen wall dorsal and ventral to the rumenostomy (see **Fig. 7**C). While the stay sutures are held in traction, the rumen wall is incised and the rumenostomy site is removed (see **Fig. 7**D). The rumen wall is then closed with

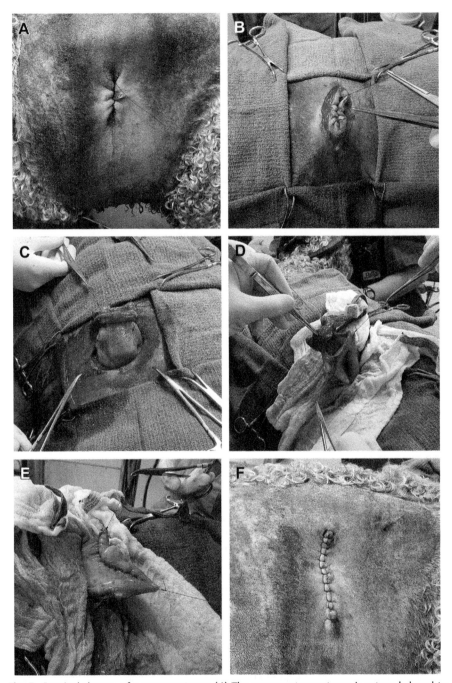

Fig. 7. Surgical closure of a rumenostomy. (*A*) The rumenostomy stoma is sutured closed to minimize leakage and contamination while performing the procedure. (*B*) The skin and muscle layers are incised around the rumenostomy stoma while it is held in tension with stay sutures. (*C*) The rumenostomy is exteriorized and stay sutures are placed in the rumen wall to facilitate resection of the rumenostomy while keeping the open rumen wall exteriorized from the abdominal cavity. (*D*) The rumen wall is incised to remove the rumenostomy site. (*E*) The rumen is closed with a double-layer simple continuous suture followed by a Cushing pattern of absorbable suture. (*F*) The body wall and skin are closed.

absorbable suture in 2 layers with a simple continuous pattern followed by a Cushing pattern (see **Fig. 7**E). The muscle wall and skin are then closed in routine fashion for a laparotomy (see **Fig. 7**F).

SUMMARY

Temporary rumenostomy is a useful procedure for the treatment, management, and support of patients with forestomach disease of various types. The rumenostomy provides a mechanism for relief of chronic rumen tympany or distention, removal of rumen contents and lavage of the rumen, removal of some rumen foreign bodies, administration of rumen fluid transfaunation, and administration of enteral nutrition or other medications. When the rumenostomy is no longer necessary, it can be allowed to close by second intention or by surgical resection.

REFERENCES

1. Walker W. Surgery of the ruminant forestomach compartments. In: Fubini SL, Ducharme NG, editors. Farm animal surgery. 2nd edition. St Louis (MO): Elsevier; 2017. p. 249–60.
2. Lozier JW, Niehaus AJ. Surgery of the forestomach. Vet Clin North Am Food Anim Pract 2016;32(3):617–28.
3. Laflin SL, Gnad DP. Rumen cannulation: procedure and use of a cannulated bovine. Vet Clin North Am Food Anim Pract 2008;24(2):335–40, vii.
4. Hartnack AK, Niehaus AJ, Rousseau M, et al. Indications for and factors relating to outcome after rumenotomy or rumenostomy in cattle: 95 cases (1999-2011). J Am Vet Med Assoc 2015;247(6):659–64.
5. Garry F, McConnel C. Indigestion in ruminants. In: Smith BP, editor. Large animal internal medicine. 5th edition. St Louis (MO): Elsevier; 2015. p. 777–99.
6. DePeters EJ, George LW. Rumen transfaunation. Immunol Lett 2014;162(2 Pt A): 69–76.
7. Shakespeare AS. Rumen management during aphagia. J S Afr Vet Assoc 2008; 79(3):106–12.
8. Chigerwe M, Tyler JW, Dawes ME, et al. Enteral feeding of 3 mature cows by rumenostomy. J Vet Intern Med 2005;19(5):779–81.
9. Franz S, Gentile A, Baumgartner W. Comparison of two ruminoscopy techniques in calves. Vet J 2006;172(2):308–14.
10. Pearson EG, Guard CL, Smith DF. A method for obtaining abomasal fluid via a rumen fistula. Cornell Vet 1981;71(2):183–7.
11. Noordsy JL. Treating chronic ruminal tympany with a temporary ruminal fistula. CompContEd Pract Vet 1997;19(11):1306–16.
12. Edmondson MA. Local, regional, and spinal anesthesia in ruminants. Vet Clin North Am Food Anim Pract 2016;32(3):535–52.
13. Jasmin BH, Boston RC, Modesto RB, et al. Perioperative ruminal pH changes in domestic sheep (*Ovis aries*) housed in a biomedical research setting. J Am Assoc Lab Anim Sci 2011;50(1):27–32.
14. Rager KD, George LW, House JK, et al. Evaluation of rumen transfaunation after surgical correction of left-sided displacement of the abomasum in cows. J Am Vet Med Assoc 2004;225(6):915–20.

Rumen Microbiome, Probiotics, and Fermentation Additives

Joshua C. McCann, PhD*, Ahmed A. Elolimy, MS,
Juan J. Loor, PhD*

KEYWORDS

- Rumen • Nutrition • Metabolism • Digestion • Probiotics • Fermentation

KEY POINTS

- The role of ruminal microorganisms (bacteria, protozoa, fungi, archaea, and viruses) in the breakdown and use of feedstuffs through fermentation has been long recognized.
- End products of fermentation along with microbial mass provide sources of energy and substrates for the synthesis of lipid, glucose, and protein by the animal.
- Rumen microorganisms play an essential role in optimizing nutrient use from feed.
- Rapid advances in phylogenetics and the development of high-throughput sequencing tools have advanced our knowledge of the ecology and functional capacity of ruminal microbial ecosystems.
- Application of omics tools in the evaluation of manipulators of ruminal fermentation can provide added value when optimizing feedstuff and minimizing digestive disorders.

INTRODUCTION
Significance of the Ruminal Microbiome

Hungate's seminal book on "The Rumen and Its Microbes" was paramount not only in detailing the progress in the field during the 25 years before 1966, but also because it provided a framework for the potential application of basic rumen microbial biology in the context of agricultural applications.[1] The "Introduction" chapter of Hungate's book provides a fascinating historical account about written evidence going back to Leviticus, demonstrating that ruminant animals were distinguished from their mammalian counterparts. In a series of classic reviews published in 1983,[2,3] authors had at their disposal well over 2000 peer-reviewed articles dealing with various aspects of ruminal digestion, for example, nitrogen and carbohydrate metabolism along with the fermentation pathways and the major microbial species. The millions of

Disclosure Statement: The authors have nothing to disclose.
Department of Animal Sciences, Division of Nutritional Sciences, University of Illinois, 1207 West Gregory Drive, Urbana, IL 61801, USA
* Corresponding authors.
E-mail addresses: jcmccan2@illinois.edu (J.C.M.); jloor@illinois.edu (J.J.L.)

microorganisms harbored in the reticulorumen include bacteria, archea, viruses, fungi, and protozoa. These microbial communities can produce a wide array of enzymes with essential roles in the breakdown of plant lignocellulosic and nonstructural carbohydrate (starch, sugars), nitrogenous compounds (plant protein, amino acids, urea), and lipids.[4]

From a quantitative standpoint, the process of ruminal fermentation of carbohydrate to produce the volatile fatty acids (VFA) is central not only for ensuring availability of energy (ATP) for microbial growth but also to provide the animal with the molecules that are essential to produce glucose (gluconeogenesis), lipid (acetate, butyrate), and energy-releasing fuels (acetate, butyrate). Microbial metabolism of nitrogen-containing compounds is also central to the microbial economy, because it provides the backbones for synthesis of microbial protein that in turn serves a source of amino acids for protein accretion (muscle, milk) in the animal.[5] The interrelationship between carbohydrate and protein–nitrogen metabolism by the ruminal microbes, also described as "nutrient synchrony," has been the subject of substantial research since the 1970s.[6] Clearly, ruminal microorganisms play an essential role in optimizing nutrient use from feed. The fact that feedstuffs and feed additives commonly fed to ruminants alter the microbial ecology of the rumen has allowed nutritionists to explore management strategies to optimize further not only the capture of nutrients by the microbiota and the host, but also to manipulate the balance and activities of microbes in the rumen (probiotics, prebiotics).[7]

By the 1990s and before the rise of the 'omics' approaches (eg, high-throughput sequencing), implementation of classical culture approaches was paramount in enhancing our understanding of the rumen microbial ecology and the nutrition of microorganisms. At least 22 major bacteria had been characterized by the beginning of the 21st century.[4] Rapid technical advances in the last 10 years have allowed the identification of the composition, structure, diversity, and function of microbial ecosystems in the rumen.[8] These advances have enabled scientists, for the first time, to have a holistic view of the rumen microbiota. The present review has been divided into sections concerned with (1) technology for microbial research, (2) importance of ruminal manipulation, and (3) manipulators of ruminal fermentation. Manipulators of ruminal fermentation are further subdivided into probiotics (bacteria, live yeast, and fungi), and fermentation additives (yeast, secondary plant metabolites, enzymes, and ionophores) (**Table 1**).

TECHNOLOGY FOR MICROBIAL RESEARCH: THEN, NOW, AND TOMORROW

The first rumen microbiologists were true pioneers as they laid the foundation for our understanding of how anaerobic microbiota function.[9] From the use of the Hungate "roll-tube technique," to the continued refinement of culture media for isolation to rumen bacteria, most of the knowledge gained on rumen microbial communities has been intertwined with advances in methodology and technology.[10,11] Although the rumen is no longer one of the most popular microbial communities of interest, continued technological development remains the primary driver as our understanding of the rumen is consistently altered and redefined.[8]

The field of microbiology began evolving into culture independent techniques in the early 1990s. No longer were scientist limited to the species they could isolate from a community. Some of the first nucleic acid-based techniques were used to study the rumen and included polymerase chain reaction and community fingerprinting strategies such as denatured gradient gel electrophoresis, restriction fragment length polymorphism, and automated ribosomal intergenic spacer analysis. Sanger sequencing

Table 1
Examples of feed additive supplementation in ruminant nutrition

Product	Manufacturer	Product Details	Supplementation	Main Effects	Animal Model and Reference
Diamond-V XP yeast culture	Diamond-V (USA)	*Saccharomyces cerevisiae*	57 g/d/head	↑ DM and protein digestion ↑ propionate production ↓ microbial protein	Lactating cows and in vitro[60]
A-Max yeast culture concentrate	Vi-Cor (USA)	*S cerevisiae*	57 g/d/head	↑ DM and protein digestion ↑ propionate % ↑ rumen pH ↑ microbial nitrogen digestion	Lactating cows and in vitro[60]
BIOSAF SC 47	Lesaffre Feed Additives (France)	*S cerevisiae Sc47*	5 g/d/head	↑ VFA concentrations and rumen pH ↑ fibrolytic and lactate-using bacteria	Early lactating cows[25]
Actisaf Sc 47	Lesaffre Feed Additives (France)	*S cerevisiae*	10 g/d/head	↓ acetate:propionate ratio ↓ Bacteroidetes, ↑Fibrobacter bacteria	Mid-to-late lactating cows[7]
Fungi					
Orpinomyces strain KNGF-2	Locally isolated in the laboratory	Isolated from the rumen of Korean native black goats	200 mL/head	↑ nutrient digestibility and nitrogen retention ↑ bacteria and fungi abundance	Mature sheep[61]
Orpinomyces sp. C-14 and *Piromyces* sp. WNG-12	National Dairy Research Institute (India)	*Orpinomyces* sp. C-14 and *Piromyces* sp. WNG-12 broth culture	160 mL/d/head for buffalo calves 250 mL/wk/head for lactating buffaloes	↑ digestibility of DM, crude protein, NDF, ADF and cellulose ↑production of VFA, total nitrogen and trichloroacid precipitable nitrogen ↓ ruminal pH and ammonia nitrogen ↑ zoospores	Buffalo calves and lactating buffaloes[28,30]

(continued on next page)

Table 1
(continued)

Product	Manufacturer	Product Details	Supplementation	Main Effects	Animal Model and Reference
Yeast products					
MTB-100	Alltech (USA)	Yeast-derived cell wall preparation	20, 40, or 60 g/d/head	↓ ruminal indigestible ADF outflow and liquid dilution rate; ↓ fescue toxicosis	Beef steers and cows[37]
Diamond V XP Yeast Culture	Diamond V (USA)	S cerevisiae fermentation product	56 g/d/head	↔ rumen microbial populations	Lactating cows[35]
TruMax	Vi-COR (USA)	Enzymatically hydrolyzed yeast cell wall	1, 2, or 3 g enzymatically hydrolyzed yeast cell wall/head/d	↓ acetate:propionate ratio and methane emissions; ↑ propionate proportion	Holstein steers[38]
Solid powder	Diamond V (USA)	S cerevisiae fermentation product	6 g/kg DMI	↓ ruminal ammonia nitrogen; ↓ methane emissions; ↔ diversity and copy number of methanogens	Growing goats[34]
Tannins					
Condensed tannins from Lotus corniculatus	Grazing L corniculatus pasture	Condensed tannins	Sheep were grazed outdoors on L corniculatus pasture	↓ proteolytic rumen bacteria population such as Clostridium proteoclasticum B316T, Butyrivibrio fibrisolvens C211a, Eubacterium sp. C12b, and Streptococcus bovis B315; ↔ rumen microbial protein in the rumen and microbial protein outflow from the rumen to the abomasum	Sheep[49]
Rain tree (Samanea saman) pod meal	Locally harvested and prepared	Crude tannins and saponins	60 g/kg of total DMI	↑ Fibrobacter succinogenes; ↓ ruminal protozoa and methanogen	Dairy steers[50]

Pistachio byproducts extract	Locally prepared pistachio byproducts extract	Tannic acid as pistachio byproducts extract	1% tannic acid on DM basis	↓ ruminal ammonia nitrogen and microbial nitrogen synthesis ↔ microbial nitrogen supply	Dairy goat[47]
Silvafeed ByPro	Silvateam (Italy)	Quebracho tannin extract	15 or 30 g quebracho tannin extract/kg DM of diet	↓ fiber digestion and nitrogen apparent total tract digestibility ↓ ruminal degradation of dietary protein, apparent total tract digestibility of dry matter and organic matter (30 g/kg level) ↓ microbial protein production in the rumen	Dairy cows[62]
Indusol ATO	Otto Dille (Germany)	Quebracho tannin extract from the heartwood of the quebracho tree (*Schinopsis lorentzii* [Griseb.] Griseb. and *Schinopsis balansae* Engl.)	1%, 2%, 4%, or 6% Quebracho tannin extract on DM basis	↑ propionate and butyrate proportions (liner dose response) ↓ acetate, isobutyrate and isovalerate proportions (linear dose) ↓ rumen fermentation and microbial biomass yields (at low and moderate doses)	Nonlactating heifers[63]
Extract of the Quebracho plant (*Schinopsis balansae*)	Commercial product	Condensed tannins	1%, 2%, 3% and 4%/kg DM	↓ methane emissions ↔ nitrogen balance or ruminal microbial protein production	Heifers[64]
Tannic acid	Sinopharm Chemical Reagent Company (China)	Tannic acid (purity 99.9%)	26 g/kg DM	↓ DM, organic matter and crude protein digestibility ↓ VFA production, acetate:propionate, ammonia nitrogen and methane emissions ↓ protozoa, methanogens and *Ruminococcus albus*	Male beef cattle[52]

Abbreviations: ADF, acid detergent fiber; DM, dry matter; DMI, dry matter intake; NDF, neutral detergent fiber; VFA, volatile fatty acids.

and library building using plasmids and cloning vectors were used to describe genes of interest and for the first bacterial genome assemblies. Real-time quantitative polymerase chain reaction technology facilitated greater sensitivity to detect an individual species and monitor population changes. These technologies made significant improvements in our understanding of microbial communities. However, the advent of massively paralleled, high-throughput DNA sequencing has arguably made the greatest impact of culture independent techniques and led to the creation of the term "microbiome," which refers to the microorganisms and their genomes in a given environment. Initially referred to as next-generation sequencing, it was capable of generating thousands and then millions of short reads in a single run. Barcoding individual samples with a unique identifier allowed many samples to be multiplexed within a single run, greatly reducing the costs per sample and increasing the interest in the field. By sequencing amplicons of the conserved 16S rRNA gene, the taxonomy of observed bacteria can be determined at the phylum to species level. Although Roche/454 sequencers initially were the most common platform initially, the greater throughput of Illumina's HiSeq and MiSeq platforms has made them the most popular for microbiome and metagenome research. A third generation of sequencing platforms has also been developed by Oxford Nanopore and Pacific Biosciences, which generate longer reads and require no amplification during sequencing to reduce bias of short read lengths.[12] Researchers have just started to use these platforms for microbiome research and their use will likely increase as the technology continues to mature.[13–15] A more in-depth discussion on the technology advancement and current sequencing strategies can be found in an excellent review by Vincent and colleagues.[16]

Amplicon sequencing of the 16S rRNA gene is the most commonly used strategy to study the rumen microbiome compared with shotgun sequencing. Despite its recent popularity, there are many potential pitfalls in microbiome studies, including sample collection, DNA extraction bias, primer selection, chimeric sequences, operational taxonomic unit cutoffs, taxonomic assignments, and statistical methodology. The number of rumen metagenome and metatranscriptome studies is growing, but widespread adoption of these techniques is currently limited by higher costs and the required bioinformatics skills to analyze the data. Future technologies will likely fill the current technology niche between 16S rRNA amplicon sequencing and shotgun metagenomics to allow a more refined description of microbial communities. There has been a committed effort to sequence the genomes of ruminal bacteria and archaea by the Hungate 1000 project, but it is widely accepted that there remain many uncultured rumen bacteria. Future technologies will also advance our understanding of how microbial communities function cooperatively using assembled mock community and systems biology approaches.

IMPORTANCE OF RUMINAL MANIPULATION

Ruminants have classically been considered very efficient owing to their ability to convert low-quality and unusable feedstuffs into nutritionally dense, consumable meat and milk. Maintaining proper rumen fermentation is critical for ruminants to preserve their modern ecological niche. Although cattle are often critiqued for their low feed efficiency compared with swine and poultry, a substantially greater proportion of feedstuffs consumed by cattle are not edible by humans, such as forage, distillers grains, and many other industrial coproducts. Regardless, ruminal degradation of fiber is the least efficient aspect of digestion for ruminants and may conflict with other nutritionally influenced demands of production. Thus, manipulation of the rumen can often lead to greater animal performance, profitability, and overall sustainability of cattle systems.

MANIPULATORS OF RUMINAL FERMENTATION
Probiotics

Supplemental bacteria

Although many bacteria have been isolated from the rumen and other gut environments, there are limited examples of reintroducing a selected isolate into the rumen with any residual persistence. The success of adding a bacterial species to the rumen is largely dictated by the availability of a niche a given bacterium would fill.[17] All bacteria and microbes present in a community occupy or share an ecological niche. The competitiveness of a niche is related to the prevalence of that function among community members and determines the likelihood of persistence in vivo. Thus, the expected persistence of dosing a fibrolytic bacterium would be decreased compared with a lactate-using bacterium or other specialized functions. A recent review of the literature supports this generalization and contains a further description of the challenges that exist for an introduced strain.[17]

Specialized or unoccupied niches within the rumen offer the greatest opportunity for persistence of a dosed bacterium. *Leucaena leucocephala*, a tropical legume, contains high levels of mimosine, a nonprotein amino acid. Some goats were sensitive to mimosine poisoning, but transferring ruminal contents from resistant goats successfully conferred resistance to the once susceptible goats.[18] Later, the responsible novel species, *Synergistes jonesii*, was isolated and notably mimosine was one of only a few identified growth substrates.[19] The lactate-using bacteria, *Megasphaera elsdenii*, is commonly observed within the rumen, but often at very low levels. Given the role of lactate in the onset of acute and subacute ruminal acidosis (SARA), reduced lactate levels are often linked with greater animal production and fiber degradation. Dosing of selected *M elsdenii* strains has proved useful in further reducing the prevalence of acidosis.[20] Other commercial probiotics include lactic acid–producing bacteria as a means of maintaining more consistent populations of lactate users to prevent acidotic bouts. However, research is limited in this area for the effectiveness of this strategy.

Live yeast

Live yeast cells have the potential to play a dual probiotic–prebiotic active role in the rumen. The probiotic action of the yeast can be explained through modulating the composition and activities of the rumen microbial ecosystem, leading to a decrease in lactic acid content, an increase and maintenance of ruminal pH, an improvement in nutrient digestibility, an optimization of VFA profiles, and a decrease in ruminal ammonia production.[21] Another positive effect of dietary yeast is to alter ruminal fermentation to reduce methane production, consequently decreasing energy losses during fermentation.[22] Although yeasts are aerobic microbes, they have oxygen-scavenging properties to maintain an anaerobic environment required for optimal fermentation.[23] In addition, direct-fed yeast cells elicit a prebiotic effect through compounds such as oligosaccharides, amino acids, vitamins, and organic acids contained within yeast cells, all of which can stimulate microbial communities in the rumen to grow.[24] Therefore, dietary yeast can have a beneficial effect on ruminal efficiency.

The most commonly used strain of yeast in ruminant nutrition is *Saccharomyces cerevisiae*, which can help to stabilize ruminal pH to activate fiber-degrading bacteria in the rumen, leading to improved fiber digestibility. To confirm this hypothesis, Pinloche and colleagues[25] applied pyrosequencing to uncover changes in ruminal bacteria in response to active dry yeast supplementation to early lactation dairy cows. Results indicated that lactate-using bacteria (eg, *Megasphaera* and *Selenomonas*) had higher abundance, thus confirming the role of yeast in decreasing lactic acid concentration and helping maintain normal ruminal pH. Yeast supplementation also increased the relative abundance of fibrolytic-degrading bacteria such as *Fibrobacter* and *Ruminococcus*, which would enhance fiber digestion in the rumen. These findings are in accordance with observations reported more recently by Uyeno and colleagues,[26] who determined that supplementing midlactation dairy cows with 10 g of active yeast cells on a daily basis for 21 days activated fibrolytic bacteria in the rumen.

From a quantitative standpoint, supplementing diets with yeast increases dry matter (DM) digestion, protein use, total VFA and propionate production, and decreases the acetate to propionate ratio, and ammonia and methane release in dairy cows and growing goats.[26] Most of these studies focused on the effects of dietary supplemental *S cerevisiae*, but little is known about the effect of other yeast species on ruminal fermentation. For instance, Wang and colleagues[21] compared the effects of different yeast strains (*S cerevisiae*, *Candida tropicalis*, and *Candida utilis*) on maize stover and rice straw digestion in vitro. Results indicated that *C tropicalis* was the only one to improve fermentation as indicated by the greater disappearance of DM and neutral detergent fiber, along with lower methane production.

Modern intensive beef and dairy production systems require stimulating fast muscle growth and high milk production, respectively, by feeding ruminants diets of high ruminal fermentability, which increase the risk of metabolic disorders, for example, SARA and acidosis. These disorders are associated with an imbalance of the ruminal microbial ecosystem, all of which perturb the normal functioning of the rumen, eventually causing a reduction in feed intake, poor health, and low productivity. Therefore, incorporation of yeast supplementation in ruminant diets could be a practical means for maintaining normal rumen function and overall animal health. The positive effects on digestibility of high forage diets also underscore the potential for yeast supplementation to optimize the use of lower quality feeds.

Fungi-based feed supplementation

Fungi supplementation can elicit a "fibrolytic effect" in the rumen by colonizing and physically disrupting plant fractions to increase the access of fiber surfaces for bacteria and their fiber-degrading enzymes.[27] By increasing the abundance of rumen fungi, its supplementation could enhance ammonia use during fermentation. In turn, these effects may enhance bacterial growth and increase microbial protein production.[28] Fungi also can produce a wide array of cellulolytic and hemicellulolytic enzymes to break down lignin and hemicellulose,[29] which could enhance nutrient digestibility of fibrous feeds.

The total fungi and cellulolytic bacterial biomass in the rumen increases with direct-fed fungi.[28] As a result, cellulolytic (carboxymethylcellulase) and xylanolytic (xylanase) activities are increased leading to overall benefits in the digestibility of crude protein, cellulose, neutral detergent fiber, and acid detergent fiber and consequently the total production of VFA.[30,31] Such responses help to explain the better use of fibrous feeds and the increase in VFA concentration and microbial protein production with dietary fungi. These microorganisms also have the capacity to increase numbers of lactate-using bacteria such as *Selenomonas ruminantium* and *M elsdenii*,[32] which would be important in decreasing the susceptibility to SARA or ruminal acidosis particularly when high-grain or high-concentrate diets are fed. Fungi also play a role in inhibiting the growth and activity of methanogens[33]; therefore, dietary fungi can decrease feed energy losses and increase energy supply for growth and production.

From a practical standpoint, most of the available pieces of evidence indicate that fungal supplementation has promise particularly when high-producing cattle are fed diets containing rapidly fermentable carbohydrates, for example, early lactation dairy cows and finishing beef cattle. Those animals are at higher risk of developing acidosis and SARA. In addition, the fact that dietary fungi improve the digestibility of high-forage and poor-quality diets is indicative of added benefits in terms of performance.[33]

FERMENTATION ADDITIVES
Yeast Products

Yeast cell wall, a yeast product, has the potential to be used as a prebiotic in ruminant nutrition for its positive effects on fermentation activities in the rumen. The few studies available on yeast cell wall indicate that rumen health and fermentation respond in the same way as the rumen reacts to supplemental live yeast in terms of improving fiber digestion, decreasing acetate to propionate molar ratio and reducing methane production. Yeast fermentation products are also used in animal nutrition as a prebiotic. For example, providing dietary S cerevisiae fermentation products decreased ruminal ammonia concentration and reduced methane emissions, but surprisingly did not change the relative abundance of ruminal methanogens.[34,35] Furthermore, adding S cerevisiae fermentation products to lactating Holstein cow diets improved rumen health and digestive function.[36]

To our knowledge, there are no published studies investigating changes in rumen microbial ecology to supplementing ruminant diets with yeast cell wall. Some of the in vivo fermentation data also are not consistent with in vitro work. For instance, available results from in vitro studies indicated a positive response of yeast cell wall supplementation on fermentation activities in terms of increasing fiber degradation and altering VFA profile as indicated by lower proportions of acetate, higher propionate, and lower acetate to propionate ratio.[37,38] Therefore, it seems that yeast cell walls may elicit the same effects as supplementing live yeast. Accordingly, yeast cell wall would stimulate the growth and proliferation of cellulolytic microbial communities in the rumen, but this hypothesis remains to be verified. In contrast, feeding goats or lactating dairy cows with S cerevisiae fermentation products did not affect the composition of bacterial communities in the rumen, including methanogens.[34,35]

In studies conducted by Merrill and colleagues[37] and Salinas-Chavira and colleagues,[38] supplementing yeast cell wall to beef cattle revealed a potential for beneficial effects on the rumen. For example, finishing feedlot steers fed enzymatically hydrolyzed yeast cells for 229 days increased DM intake and enhanced average daily gain. This response was associated with better fiber degradation in the rumen and a lower acetate to propionate ratio.[38] Also, feeding steers with yeast-derived cell wall for 29 days stimulated fiber digestion in the rumen through decreasing indigestible acid detergent fiber outflow from the rumen.[37] Supplementing yeast-derived cell wall to Angus × Hereford lactating cows fed high alkaloid tall fescue increased serum prolactin after calving, which the authors argued could be a beneficial effect of the yeast through a decrease in the severity of fescue toxicosis.[37] Overall, these results are in line with the effects of supplementation of yeast cells (see the Yeast section).

Supplementing S cerevisiae fermentation products to growing goats at the rate of 6 or 12 g/kg DM intake did not alter the digestibility of organic matter, neutral detergent fiber, or acid detergent fiber.[34] In addition, S cerevisiae fermentation products decreased ruminal ammonia production and methane emissions in vivo.[34] In another study, compared with lactating Holstein cows consuming less than 26 kg DM/d, providing 56 g of S cerevisiae fermentation product per day to cows consuming more than 26 kg DM/d helped to maintain ruminal pH in part by reducing the true and apparent ruminal starch digestibility.[39] Therefore, in the long-term, *S cerevisiae* supplementation to high-producing cows could help to reduce the likelihood of SARA. Through increasing microbial protein and fiber-degrading fungi in the rumen, fermentation products of *S cerevisiae* also improved in vitro digestibility of forage (such as rice straw, corn stover, or corn silage with or without grain) and corn–soybean meal–based diets supplemented with corn stover, corn silage, and alfalfa.[40]

The available few studies on the potential effects of supplementing hydrolyzed yeast cell wall to cattle formulas indicate a promising role for dietary yeast cell wall on improving forage use by optimizing ruminal VFA profiles in the same way as dietary yeast cells. *S cerevisiae* fermentation products also can be added to high-starch dairy diets to help stabilize ruminal pH through controlling ruminal starch digestibility. As such, the potential risks of digestive disorders associated with feeding high-starch diets would be minimized.

Plant Secondary Metabolites

Nutritionists have for a long time considered plant secondary metabolites (tannins, flavonoids, and saponnins) as antinutritional factors owing to their detrimental effects on feed intake, nutrient use, animal productivity, and health.[41] However, recent research has indicated that the negative or positive effects of secondary metabolites depend on their origin, chemical composition, dietary concentration, and feed quality. Therefore, findings obtained from numerous in vivo and in vitro studies with cattle, sheep, and goats recommend incorporating limited amounts of secondary metabolites into diets to improve feed use. These compounds are expected to have a positive impact on animal performance by enhancing ruminal fermentation, shifting the ruminal microbial ecosystem to contain fewer methane-producing microorganisms, reducing excessive dietary protein degradation, and inducing microbial protein production.[42–44]

Tannins are one of the most extensively studied secondary plant metabolites in animal nutrition. Tannins are polymers of phenolic compounds with various molecular weights and chemical structures found in plants.[45] These compounds are capable of protecting dietary proteins from rapid and excessive degradation in the rumen by forming insoluble tannin–protein complexes, which reduce dietary protein breakdown.[46] As a result, less ammonia is produced, nitrogen loss from dietary protein decreases, and the flow of amino acids to the small intestine increases.[47] Therefore, supplemental tannins can enhance the efficiency of dietary protein use by increasing the flow of amino acids to the small intestine.

The reduction of protein degradation in the rumen when tannins are supplemented to animal feeds occurs as a result of decreasing ruminal proteolytic bacterial populations such as *Clostridium proteoclasticum*, *Butyrivibrio fibrisolvens*, *Eubacterium* sp., and *Streptococcus bovis*.[48–50] Tannins could mitigate methane emissions by decreasing the growth of predominant methanogenic bacteria, protozoa, and archaea.[51,52] Such an effect would reduce energy losses and allow more available energy and protein for animal use. In addition, the stimulation of ruminal biohydrogenation of polyunsaturated fatty acids observed when tannins are supplemented in vitro generates greater amounts of *trans*11-18:1 and *cis*9,*trans*11-18:2 fatty acids, both of which are considered to be beneficial for human health.[45] Therefore, the role of tannins in ruminant diets goes beyond ruminal protein metabolism. Overall, the positive effect of dietary tannin supplementation is through direct impacts on rumen microbes and their metabolism.

Dietary tannins have the ability to prevent bloating, which is a serious digestive disorder that occurs when dietary proteins are degraded rapidly in the rumen, forming a stable foam that traps ruminal gases, inhibits eructation, causes severe pain, reduces production efficiency, and may result in animal death.[48,53] Owing to the efficiency of tannins in forming tannin–protein complexes to reduce the excessive ruminal protein degradation and decrease methane production, supplemental tannins play a key role in controlling the incidence of bloat in ruminants.

Ionophores

Despite their original intention as a coccidostat, ionophore antibiotics have been arguably the most successful feed additive used in ruminant production for 40 years. Although feeding ionophores has shown to be effective in many production settings, their use is especially widespread in the beef feedlot industry. However, ionophores remain underused in grazing conditions. Ionophores approved for use in animal production include monensin, lasalocid, laidlomycin, and salinomycin.[54] The response of feeding ionophores to ruminants is well-documented and varies slightly depending on the compound. Overall, ionophores decrease feed intake without reducing growth to improve feed conversion. The feed efficiency benefits result from increasing energy and nitrogen metabolism and hindering the occurrence of digestive disorders.[55]

The efficacy of ionophores is rooted in alterations to rumen microbiota. Although ionophores primarily affect gram-positive bacteria, exceptions suggest additional cell membrane structures or mechanisms determine susceptibility and intrinsic resistance. Ionophores bind to cations to facilitate their transfer across the cell membrane, which disrupts the proton gradient leading to energy spilling and limited growth.[54] The most notable bacteria reduced by ionophores include H_2 producers, NH_3 producers, and lactate producers.[56] The resulting impact on ruminal fermentation is greater propionate:acetate ratio, protein availability, and ruminal pH.[56] By decreasing the accumulation of H_2 from protozoa, substrates for methanogenesis are limited and thus reduce methane production.[56,57] Increasing ruminal pH decreases the occurrence of acidosis in feedlot cattle and improves overall performance.[58,59] Although the efficacy of ionophores has been demonstrated, their classification as an antibiotic may put their future use at risk despite no relevance to human medicine.

SUMMARY

The rumen is a highly adaptive, diverse, and competitive microbial environment in a constant state of flux even within a single day. However, the possibility of improving rumen function still exists and attempts to alter ruminal fermentation using feed additives and probiotics have been made for many years. Motivations for ruminal manipulation are rooted in a desire to make incremental, positive changes to optimize fermentation, and subsequently performance without occurrence of digestive disorders. Historical and current challenges in ruminant production profitability have contributed to the desire to improve rumen function and fermentation. In addition, some countries have eliminated the use of several older technologies renewing demand for a new generation of products. For example, feed grade antibiotics are not permitted in various countries around the world. Further restrictions on the use of growth promotants, including hormonal implants and beta-agonists, has increased the attention and research to improve ruminant production via rumen function optimization to recover production losses for elimination of older, more proven technologies. The advent of technology to study at a large scale not only the ecology of microorganisms in the rumen, but also their functional capacity in the context of digestive function has greatly advanced our fundamental knowledge of this ecosystem. These technologies have already been used in evaluating different feed additives that could aid in manipulating the ruminal ecosystem for the benefit of cattle, particularly within intensive management systems such as dairy and beef cattle production.

REFERENCES

1. Friedrichs P, Saremi B, Winand S, et al. Energy and metabolic sensing G protein-coupled receptors during lactation-induced changes in energy balance. Domest Anim Endocrinol 2014;48:33–41.
2. Baldwin RL, Allison MJ. Rumen metabolism. J Anim Sci 1983;57(Suppl 2): 461–77.
3. Owens FN, Bergen WG. Nitrogen metabolism of ruminant animals: historical perspective, current understanding and future implications. J Anim Sci 1983; 57(Suppl 2):498–518.
4. Russell JB, Rychlik JL. Factors that alter rumen microbial ecology. Science 2001; 292(5519):1119–22.
5. Bach A, Calsamiglia S, Stern MD. Nitrogen metabolism in the rumen. J Dairy Sci 2005;88(Suppl 1):E9–21.
6. Hall MB, Huntington GB. Nutrient synchrony: sound in theory, elusive in practice. J Anim Sci 2008;86(14 Suppl):E287–92.
7. Uyeno Y, Shigemori S, Shimosato T. Effect of probiotics/prebiotics on cattle health and productivity. Microbes Environ 2015;30(2):126–32.
8. McCann JC, Wickersham TA, Loor JJ. High-throughput methods redefine the rumen microbiome and its relationship with nutrition and metabolism. Bioinform Biol Insights 2014;8:109–25.
9. Krause DO, Nagaraja TG, Wright ADG, et al. Board-invited review: rumen microbiology: leading the way in microbial ecology. J Anim Sci 2013;91(1):331–41.
10. Hungate RE. A roll tube method for cultivation of strict aneraobes. In: Norris JR, Ribbons DW, editors. Methods in Microbiology. Cambridge (MA): Academic Press; 1969. p. 117–32.
11. Kenters N, Henderson G, Jeyanathan J, et al. Isolation of previously uncultured rumen bacteria by dilution to extinction using a new liquid culture medium. J Microbiol Methods 2011;84(1):52–60.
12. Bleidorn C. Third generation sequencing: technology and its potential impact on evolutionary biodiversity research. Syst Biodivers 2016;14(1):1–8.
13. Wagner J, Coupland P, Browne HP, et al. Evaluation of PacBio sequencing for full-length bacterial 16S rRNA gene classification. BMC Microbiol 2016;16(1):274.
14. Schloss PD, Jenior ML, Koumpouras CC, et al. Sequencing 16S rRNA gene fragments using the PacBio SMRT DNA sequencing system. PeerJ 2016;4:e1869.
15. White Iii RA, Callister SJ, Moore RJ, et al. The past, present and future of microbiome analyses. Nat Protoc 2016;11(11):2049–53.
16. Vincent AT, Derome N, Boyle B, et al. Next-generation sequencing (NGS) in the microbiological world: how to make the most of your money. J Microbiol Methods 2017;138:60–71.
17. Weimer PJ. Redundancy, resilience and host specificity of the ruminal microbiota: implications for engineering improved ruminal fermentations. Front Microbiol 2015;6:296.
18. Jones RJ, Megarrity RG. Successful transfer of DHP-degrading bacteria from Hawaiian goats to Australian ruminants to overcome the toxicity of Leucaena. Aust Vet J 1986;63(8):259–62.

19. Allison MJ, Mayberry WR, McSweeney CS, et al. Synergistes jonesii, gen. nov., sp.nov.: a rumen bacterium that degrades toxic pyridinediols. Syst Appl Microbiol 1992;15(4):522–9.

20. Meissner HH, Henning PH, Horn CH, et al. Ruminal acidosis: a review with detailed reference to the controlling agent Megasphaera elsdenii NCIMB 41125. S Afr J Anim Sci 2010;79–100.

21. Wang Z, He Z, Beauchemin KA, et al. Evaluation of different yeast species for improving in vitro fermentation of cereal straws. Asian-Australas J Anim Sci 2016;29(2):230–40.

22. Ruiz O, Castillo Y, Arzola C, et al. Effects of Candida norvegensis live cells on in vitro oat straw rumen fermentation. Asian-Australas J Anim Sci 2016;29(2):211–8.

23. Newbold CJ, Wallace RJ, McIntosh FM. Mode of action of the yeast Saccharomyces cerevisiae as a feed additive for ruminants. Br J Nutr 1996;76(2):249–61.

24. Opsi F, Fortina R, Tassone S, et al. Effects of inactivated and live cells of Saccharomyces cerevisiae on in vitro ruminal fermentation of diets with different forage:-concentrate ratio. J Agric Sci 2012;150(2):271–83.

25. Pinloche E, McEwan N, Marden JP, et al. The effects of a probiotic yeast on the bacterial diversity and population structure in the rumen of cattle. PLoS One 2013;8(7):e67824.

26. Uyeno Y, Akiyama K, Hasunuma T, et al. Effects of supplementing an active dry yeast product on rumen microbial community composition and on subsequent rumen fermentation of lactating cows in the mid-to-late lactation period. Anim Sci J 2017;88(1):119–24.

27. Dagar SS, Kumar S, Mudgil P, et al. D1/D2 domain of large-subunit ribosomal DNA for differentiation of Orpinomyces spp. Appl Environ Microbiol 2011;77(18):6722–5.

28. Saxena S, Sehgal JP, Puniya AK, et al. Effect of administration of rumen fungi on production performance of lactating buffaloes. Benef Microbes 2010;1(2):183–8.

29. Chen YC, Chen WT, Liu JC, et al. A highly active beta-glucanase from a new strain of rumen fungus Orpinomyces sp.Y102 exhibits cellobiohydrolase and cellotriohydrolase activities. Bioresour Technol 2014;170:513–21.

30. Tripathi VK, Sehgal JP, Puniya AK, et al. Effect of administration of anaerobic fungi isolated from cattle and wild blue bull (Boselaphus tragocamelus) on growth rate and fibre utilization in buffalo calves. Arch Anim Nutr 2007;61(5):416–23.

31. Paul SS, Deb SM, Punia BS, et al. Fibrolytic potential of anaerobic fungi (Piromyces sp.) isolated from wild cattle and blue bulls in pure culture and effect of their addition on in vitro fermentation of wheat straw and methane emission by rumen fluid of buffaloes. J Sci Food Agric 2010;90(7):1218–26.

32. Martin SA, Nisbet DJ. Effect of direct-fed microbials on rumen microbial fermentation. J Dairy Sci 1992;75(6):1736–44.

33. Puniya AK, Salem AZM, Kumar S, et al. Role of live microbial feed supplements with reference to anaerobic fungi in ruminant productivity: a review. J Integr Agric 2015;14(3):550–60.

34. Lu Q, Wu J, Wang M, et al. Effects of dietary addition of cellulase and a Saccharomyces cerevisiae fermentation product on nutrient digestibility, rumen fermentation and enteric methane emissions in growing goats. Arch Anim Nutr 2016;70(3):224–38.

35. Mullins CR, Mamedova LK, Carpenter AJ, et al. Analysis of rumen microbial populations in lactating dairy cattle fed diets varying in carbohydrate profiles and

Saccharomyces cerevisiae fermentation product. J Dairy Sci 2013;96(9): 5872–81.

36. Li S, Yoon I, Scott M, et al. Impact of Saccharomyces cerevisiae fermentation product and subacute ruminal acidosis on production, inflammation, and fermentation in the rumen and hindgut of dairy cows. Anim Feed Sci Technology 2016;211: 50–60.

37. Merrill ML, Bohnert DW, Harmon DL, et al. The ability of a yeast-derived cell wall preparation to minimize the toxic effects of high-ergot alkaloid tall fescue straw in beef cattle. J Anim Sci 2007;85(10):2596–605.

38. Salinas-Chavira J, Arzola C, Gonzalez-Vizcarra V, et al. Influence of feeding enzymatically hydrolyzed yeast cell wall on growth performance and digestive function of feedlot cattle during periods of elevated ambient temperature. Asian-Australas J Anim Sci 2015;28(9):1288–95.

39. Allen MS, Ying Y. Effects of Saccharomyces cerevisiae fermentation product on ruminal starch digestion are dependent upon dry matter intake for lactating cows. J Dairy Sci 2012;95(11):6591–605.

40. Mao HL, Mao HL, Wang JK, et al. Effects of Saccharomyces cerevisiae fermentation product on in vitro fermentation and microbial communities of low-quality forages and mixed diets. J Anim Sci 2013;91(7):3291–8.

41. Sarwar Gilani G, Wu Xiao C, Cockell KA. Impact of antinutritional factors in food proteins on the digestibility of protein and the bioavailability of amino acids and on protein quality. Br J Nutr 2012;108(Suppl 2):S315–32.

42. Cobellis G, Trabalza-Marinucci M, Yu Z. Critical evaluation of essential oils as rumen modifiers in ruminant nutrition: a review. Sci Total Environ 2016;545-546: 556–68.

43. Patra AK, Saxena J. A new perspective on the use of plant secondary metabolites to inhibit methanogenesis in the rumen. Phytochemistry 2010;71(11–12): 1198–222.

44. Wanapat M, Kongmun P, Poungchompu O, et al. Effects of plants containing secondary compounds and plant oils on rumen fermentation and ecology. Trop Anim Health Prod 2012;44(3):399–405.

45. Costa M, Alves SP, Cabo A, et al. Modulation of in vitro rumen biohydrogenation by Cistus ladanifer tannins compared with other tannin sources. J Sci Food Agric 2017;97(2):629–35.

46. Lorenz MM, Alkhafadji L, Stringano E, et al. Relationship between condensed tannin structures and their ability to precipitate feed proteins in the rumen. J Sci Food Agric 2014;94(5):963–8.

47. Mokhtarpour A, Naserian AA, Pourmollae F, et al. Effect of treating alfalfa silage with pistachio by-products extract on Saanen dairy goats performance and microbial nitrogen synthesis. J Anim Physiol Anim Nutr (Berl) 2016;100(4):758–67.

48. Patra AK, Saxena J. Exploitation of dietary tannins to improve rumen metabolism and ruminant nutrition. J Sci Food Agric 2011;91(1):24–37.

49. Min BR, Attwood GT, Reilly K, et al. Lotus corniculatus condensed tannins decrease in vivo populations of proteolytic bacteria and affect nitrogen metabolism in the rumen of sheep. Can J Microbiol 2002;48(10):911–21.

50. Anantasook N, Wanapat M, Cherdthong A, et al. Changes of microbial population in the rumen of dairy steers as influenced by plant containing tannins and saponins and roughage to concentrate ratio. Asian-Australas J Anim Sci 2013;26(11): 1583–91.

51. Saminathan M, Sieo CC, Gan HM, et al. Effects of condensed tannin fractions of different molecular weights on population and diversity of bovine rumen

methanogenic archaea in vitro, as determined by high-throughput sequencing. Anim Feed Sci Technology 2016;216:146–60.

52. Yang K, Wei C, Zhao GY, et al. Effects of dietary supplementing tannic acid in the ration of beef cattle on rumen fermentation, methane emission, microbial flora and nutrient digestibility. J Anim Physiol Anim Nutr (Berl) 2017;101(2):302–10.

53. Wang Y, Majak W, McAllister TA. Frothy bloat in ruminants: cause, occurrence, and mitigation strategies. Anim Feed Sci Technology 2012;172(1–2):103–14.

54. Russell JB. Rumen microbiology and its role in ruminant nutrition. Ithaca (NY): Cornell University; 2002.

55. Bergen WG, Bates DB. Ionophores: their effect on production efficiency and mode of action. J Anim Sci 1984;58(6):1465–83.

56. Russell JB, Strobel HJ. Effect of ionophores on ruminal fermentation. Appl Environ Microbiol 1989;55(1):1–6.

57. Guan H, Wittenberg KM, Ominski KH, et al. Efficacy of ionophores in cattle diets for mitigation of enteric methane1. J Anim Sci 2006;84(7):1896–906.

58. Nagaraja TG, Avery TB, Bartley EE, et al. Prevention of lactic acidosis in cattle by lasalocid or monensin. J Anim Sci 1981;53(1):206–16.

59. Erickson GE, Milton CT, Fanning KC, et al. Interaction between bunk management and monensin concentration on finishing performance, feeding behavior, and ruminal metabolism during an acidosis challenge with feedlot cattle1. J Anim Sci 2003;81(11):2869–79.

60. Miller-Webster T, Hoover WH, Holt M, et al. Influence of yeast culture on ruminal microbial metabolism in continuous culture. J Dairy Sci 2002;85(8):2009–14.

61. Lee SS, Ha JK, Cheng KJ. Influence of an anaerobic fungal culture administration on in vivo ruminal fermentation and nutrient digestion. Anim Feed Sci Technology 2000;88(3–4):201–17.

62. Henke A, Dickhoefer U, Westreicher-Kristen E, et al. Effect of dietary Quebracho tannin extract on feed intake, digestibility, excretion of urinary purine derivatives and milk production in dairy cows. Arch Anim Nutr 2017;71(1):37–53.

63. Dickhoefer U, Ahnert S, Susenbeth A. Effects of quebracho tannin extract on rumen fermentation and yield and composition of microbial mass in heifers. J Anim Sci 2016;94(4):1561–75.

64. Pineiro-Vazquez AT, Canul-Solis JR, Alayon-Gamboa JA, et al. Energy utilization, nitrogen balance and microbial protein supply in cattle fed Pennisetum purpureum and condensed tannins. J Anim Physiol Anim Nutr (Berl) 2017;101(1): 159–69.

Moving?

Printed and bound by CPI Group (UK) Ltd, Croydon, CR0 4YY

03/10/2024

01040394-0008